MAKING PEACE WITH CHRONIC PAIN

A Whole-Life Strategy

MAKING PEACE WITH CHRONIC PAIN

A WHOLE-LIFE STRATEGY

Marlene E. Hunter, M.D., F.C.F.P.(C)

BRUNNER/MAZEL, *Publishers* • New York

Library of Congress Cataloging-in-Publication Data

Hunter, Marlene E. (Marlene Elva)
    Making peace with chronic pain: a whole-life strategy / Marlene
E. Hunter.
        p.   cm.
    Includes bibliographical references and index.
    ISBN 0-87630-821-3 (paper)
    1. Chronic pain.   2. Chronic pain—Case Studies.   I. Title.
RB127.H86   1996   96-29183
616'.0472—dc20   CIP

Published by
BRUNNER/MAZEL, INC.
19 Union Square West
New York, New York 10003

Manufactured in the United States of America
10 9 8 7 6 5 4 3 2 1

for
"SAMANTHA"
and all those who also struggle with chronic pain

CONTENTS

PREFACE

The book is meant to help people gradually change their concept of chronic pain and their attitude toward it. I would hope that anybody who finds it useful would be able to dip into it, many times over, a little bit at a time, as these changes gradually evolve within.

I had wanted to call this book "The Choreography of Pain and How to Change the Dance" as the title seemed to capture what people who suffer from chronic pain go through—their lives become choreographed around that pain. In the end the title went, but the metaphor remains, because I know that you who have chronic pain will understand exactly what is meant by it.

Throughout the pages, I have included many case histories to illustrate the point which I am making. Some of these are purely hypothetical, some are composites of imaginary and actual cases, and some are straightforward examples from my practice.

In all cases, the names and other identifying personal data have been changed. Nevertheless, pain sufferers may find themselves in this book, with a different name but a recognizable history. Even the purely hypothetical cases have been based on true situations which all people involved in the treatment of chronic pain syndromes will appreciate—whether patient, therapist, or physician.

There is one special case history—that of Samantha.

Samantha's story runs throughout the book. The excerpts are taken straight from my clinical notes. She has read the manuscript and offered invaluable advice. Although Samantha does not have a chronic pain syndrome in the pure sense, because she *does* have a diagnosable cause for her pain, nevertheless pain has pervaded her life for many years. The strict definition of a chronic pain *syndrome* seems picky but is important: it is the constellation of symptoms experienced by someone who has severe pain for which 'no cause' can now be found, although there may have *been* a cause earlier.

At the end of each chapter, there are several pages which are designed to bring you, the reader, into active participation. Each chapter concludes with a page (or two) of *pertinent points* from the chapter, and pages of worksheets to assist the pain sufferer in applying the ideas to his or her own situation. Finally, at the end of the book, are a research and literature review and commentaries, and a bibliography for those of you who would like to read further.

The concepts of choreography and The Dance are, of course, metaphor. However, the day-to-day life of a person in constant pain, *does* become choreographed around that pain. Everything is experienced in the context of the pain. My intention is to lift the pain out of that usual context, wherein pain annihilates sensibility and transforms people into struggling agonizers, and offer the possibility of a different awareness.

ACKNOWLEDGMENTS

My heartfelt appreciation to "Samantha" for her insight and commentary, for proofreading the basic manuscript, and for taking me to task when I hadn't made things clear.

Also to Dr. Adrienne Hunter for her proofreading and suggestions on the final manuscript.

And, as ever, to my husband, Redner, for putting up with me.

ABOUT THE AUTHOR

Marlene E. Hunter, M.D., F.C.F.P.(C), is a family physician in West Vancouver, British Columbia. She is a past president of the Canadian Society of Clinical Hypnosis (British Columbia Division) and a fellow, as well as past president, of the American Society of Clinical Hypnosis. She gives workshops and seminars internationally and is the author of *Creative Scripts for Hypnotherapy* and *Psych Yourself In! Hypnosis and Health*. She is also the editor of *Frontiers of Hypnosis*.

MAKING PEACE WITH CHRONIC PAIN

A WHOLE-LIFE STRATEGY

CHAPTER ONE

WHAT CHRONIC PAIN IS ... AND WHAT IT IS NOT

Prelude to the Dance

Samantha is an intelligent and articulate 32-year-old with gorgeous red hair and a bright, ready smile. She is a research chemist, very respected in her field. She was referred by her family physician and I asked her how I could be of help to her.

"I have migraine headaches," she said. "I have had them for twelve years."

Although she had had headaches from time to time in her teens, it was in her early twenties that they began to intensify. The pain was now so excruciating that she felt she had reached the limit of her endurance. And it was seriously interfering with her work—she had had to give up on a very important project because, with the amount of medication she needed even to keep the pain barely tolerable, she couldn't think straight.

Early last year, she was admitted to University Hospital for two or three days, because her neurologist wanted to sort out her medication and get her on a better regime.

She was there for four months.

This is a book about pain. It is a book directed particularly toward coping with a specific kind of pain—the kind that we call "chronic pain." And, more specifically, it is a book that describes a different *approach* to the "management" of chronic pain (as we say in the professional jargon) through a new interpretation of what chronic pain is all about.

This is NOT a book about some magical way to get rid of chronic pain. If there were such magic, someone would have discovered it long before now. It is natural for someone suffering from intractable pain, and for those whose mission in life it is to help people find relief from that pain, to grasp for magic. How we wish we had some! Instead, we are left face-to-face with the fact that, once most (if not all) of the conventional ways to dissolve pain have been explored, and the pain is still there, we must discover new approaches that depend on the incredible capacity of humankind to transcend otherwise intolerable situations—our strengths and resources from deep within us.

We all have such strengths and resources. Even when life seems to have bludgeoned us into submission, there is that little spark that can ignite new spirit and resolve.

This book is about a new way to discover and use those little sparks.

Because this journey involves making new interpretations, we need to clarify some of our definitions. Reading about definitions, especially if you are living with pain and looking for some help, can be a little bit boring, so let's get it out of the way right at the start.

WHAT IS "PAIN"?

Pain is a **response.** It can sometimes be thought of as the body's way of expressing anger. If someone has been injured, we can think of the body as being angry at the injury. If there is severe infection or inflammation, the body complains loudly. We even speak of the "red, hot, ANGRY" joint of an acute arthritis flare-up.

Emotional pain can also be traced to anger—anger at intrusion or injustice, anger because of fear or frustration. The body responds to this fear, this injury, this infection, through pain.

There are two main components of pain: the physiological component and the suffering component. Of the two, the suffering component is always the hardest to bear and the hardest to treat.

The physiological component is found in the neurological pathways that carry messages of pain. The stimulus comes from whichever part of the body is affected, along the sensory nerves and up the spinal cord to that part of the brain that interprets these sensations as 'pain.' These neurological pathways are present and operating even before we are born. There is evidence that even fetuses can and do respond to a painful stimulus by withdrawing from that stimulus. The smallest babies respond to pain, and so do our oldest citizens. The awareness of pain is a talent—I use that word deliberately—that is with us throughout our lives.

The suffering component reflects the interference that pain causes in our lives. Pain **intrudes** into one's life. If such an intrusion is short-lived, it is usually relatively easy to bear. But when the intrusion lasts for prolonged periods, it becomes harder and harder for a person to accept with equanimity.

Think, for instance, of someone who has had a work-related injury. There is an initial period of time when pain seems appropriate to the victim, but after a while—after going to the doctor, and getting medication, and attending physiotherapy, and diligently doing all the exercises, and then maybe being sent to a specialist, and getting *more* medication, and doing *more* physiotherapy, and really behaving oneself, and doing everything that one has been told to do, and the pain is still there or even *worse*—the unfairness of all this begins to weigh upon the person. "Why am I not getting better?" "Why isn't all of this wonderful medical expertise helping me?" "What's *wrong*?"

Sometimes doctors and other medical people are so focused on the physiological part of the pain, and how they can offer relief to the patient, that they forget to ask about the suffering part. When I ask a patient, "Tell me how this pain intrudes into your life," I see many eyes fill with tears as they answer, "No one has ever asked me that before." Then they tell me: "I can't go for walks anymore, and I used to love to walk for hours," or "I can't pick up my grandchildren," or "I can't do my gardening—it makes me cry to look at it, so neglected," or "I can't make love with my husband—now he doesn't even ask anymore and in some ways that hurts even more."

ALL PAIN IS REAL

All pain is real. This may seem to be a self-evident statement, but I am still surprised that so many patients come to me and say that they have been told the pain is "all in my head." This is, accurately, interpreted by the patient in a very negative way, as if they are being accused of making it up or imagining it.

Such feelings exacerbate the helplessness that begins to develop in the patient with long-standing pain. I know how easy it is for a doctor or nurse or physiotherapist to become frustrated or even exasperated and "try" to educate the patient into understanding that the origins of his or her particular pain are not, or are no longer, traceable to some specific organic cause, and therefore the patient must begin to reorganize his or her thinking about that pain and find ways to cope with it more comfortably. But implying that the pain is imaginary does not achieve that purpose; it only enrages the patient. Because patients usually cannot afford to be enraged at their medical support people, they swallow their anger, pushing it far beneath the surface where it bubbles and erodes their self-esteem.

This is not helpful.

In fact, because—as we have said—one way of describing pain is that it is the body's way of *expressing* anger, such suppressed fury may make the pain much worse—and this is entirely beyond the patient's awareness. Patients only know that they feel worse than ever and that their suffering has become even more intense.

PAIN IS A DISSOCIATIVE EXPERIENCE

Jargon again.

A dissociative experience is simply one in which one part of the mind is distracted from what is going on around it, and goes off on its own little tangent. Daydreaming is a very common, very mild dissociative experience: we know where we are, but for the time being, we don't care.

A motor vehicle accident might create a more serious dissociative experience. Often people have a real amnesia for the experience, which may last for quite a period of time. On the other hand, we can be very preoccupied with some situation or problem, but nevertheless still carry on and do our jobs—that is also a very typical dissociative experience.

Generally, such experiences are quite benign, and often they are really very pleasurable.

However, just ask people who have been ill for an extended period of time and they will tell you that it is as if the illness has taken over their minds and bodies. There seems to be a separation—some part of themselves is linked to the illness or pain and the other parts are not.

Pain can be thought of as just such a dissociative experience. We can ask, "What part of us* *perceives* and *takes care of* the pain? How does that part of us do that?"

When that part of us *takes over* instead of *taking care of* us, then we have entered the arena of chronic pain and chronic pain syndromes.

Acute pain, although it may be anything from mildly to excruciatingly uncomfortable, nevertheless can be thought of as a positive pain—that is, it sends a clear message to us that something is acutely wrong, and that it needs immediate attention. Such pain can be caused by injury, inflammation, infection, or one of the degenerative diseases. The baby with red, inflamed ears, the young adult with a terrible pain in the lower right part of the abdomen, the victim of a motor vehicle accident, the skier with a dislocated hip—all these people are experiencing acute pain.

If the pain is not satisfactorily taken care of (that awful pain in the belly abates when the inflamed appendix is removed), it may go on to produce secondary characteristics. These could be due, for example, to scarring, nerve involvement, or phantom pain (after amputations), or they could be due to psychogenic factors brought on by stress and anxiety and a host of other things which we will talk about later. Often there are components from several of these roots.

This is the predicament of the person who has had a work-related injury. Despite good medical care and a cooperative and

---

*Such a 'part of us' is known, in professional language, as an 'ego-state.' I'll be talking much more about ego-states later in the book. There is nothing very mysterious about an ego-state.

intelligent patient, the pain has not only not gone away, it has worsened. And everybody begins to get a little tense.

Samantha didn't understand why she was still in the hospital and why the new drugs weren't working. She could tell that her neurologist was puzzled too. She began to get a bit uptight and she knew that would probably make things worse. She also thought that she detected some negative vibes from the nurses—almost as if she were deliberately not getting better. Before she had become this neurologist's patient, many doctors and other medical people had told her that she was going to have to change her attitude—as if the headaches were all her fault. This made her even more depressed. Sometimes she found herself thinking, "What's the use?"

She was taking an awful lot of medication. That seemed to get everybody lathered up too—but it wasn't her idea. It was the neurologist's, and she was grateful to him because at least for short periods of time she was free from pain. But what was she going to do when she got out of the hospital?

The weeks wore on.

PAIN RELIEF TECHNIQUES

Pain relief techniques may be directed either toward conscious processes or toward the subconscious part of our minds. We need both approaches to relieve pain effectively.

Those techniques, which are directed more toward the conscious part of our minds generally relieve the *physiological* part of the pain. These include medication, physical relief obtained from ice, heat, or support, information about how to move (and how and when not to), or surgical intervention. They are usually very effective and the pain is short-lived. Often they, in themselves, cure or heal the problem, or buy a little time for the body to heal itself. These are the pain relief techniques that we doctors are taught about in medical school.

Those techniques, which are aimed more towards the subconscious are more likely to relieve the *suffering* component of pain. These include ways to release muscle tension, dissociation and distraction, biofeedback, or hypnotic techniques.

We'll be talking much more about some of these approaches

later in the book. They, in themselves, are not usually thought of as "cures" but instead, as ways to help patients cope with or modify the stressors in their lives so that some of these complicating factors are less intrusive. These are the techniques that we are usually NOT taught about in medical school (although I am very pleased to say that I see this changing, at least a little bit).

Chronic Pain Syndromes

When pain takes over someone's life, a host of other complications often ensue. These may include the inability to work, family problems, depression, and/or an unrealistic preoccupation with one's health. Such a collection of symptoms comes to be known as a SYNDROME. Much of this book will address the problems that are associated with various chronic pain syndromes.

If the worker in our earlier example continued to have pain, or perhaps if it became worse, it's easy to understand how this situation could lead to a chronic pain syndrome. Then all the other factors would become more and more prominent and the stressors in turn would intensify the experience of pain—it is a true vicious cycle.

I have described pain as a *response*. We must remember that "response" includes physiological response to the causative factors that can be identified (infection, injury, inflammation, etc.) and to psychological or emotional response to the other kinds of influencing factors—the stressors of daily life. There is nothing "bad" about these psychological or emotional responses—on the contrary, they are what single us out as humans. Without such responses we would simply be automatons.

When we understand these connections, we understand the true meaning of the term *psychosomatic*—the collaboration, the inextricable weaving of mind and body. It is impossible to be ill or in pain and not have a psychological response to that—an emotional response, to describe it in another way. And it is just as impossible to be emotionally upset or psychologically affected and not have a physiological response to *that*—the adrenal glands pour out their hormones, the biochemistry in the body establishes new states of equilibrium.

All pain incites these double-barrelled changes in the mind and body of the person. When pain persists—especially when it is increasingly hard to find the reason for that persistence—the emotional/psychological response becomes more pronounced and, in turn, the body responds physiologically.

And so it continues. The pain begins to take over the sufferer's life—everything becomes choreographed around the pain. Visitors? Too much pain today, couldn't keep up a conversation. Activities? Forget it—can't even move. Doctor's appointment? What's s/he going to tell me *this* time?

This is "The Dance"—the miserable, intrusive domination of one's life by chronic pain.

PERTINENT POINTS FROM CHAPTER ONE

Pain is a **response** that **intrudes** into one's life.

There are two components to pain: the **physiological** (sensory) component and the **suffering** (emotional/psychological) component.

Pain is a **dissociative** experience—it causes us to be separated from what is going on around us.

When a collection of symptoms persists for a long time it is called **a syndrome.**

The syndrome of chronic pain **takes over** one's life: this is what I have metaphorically called **"The Dance."**

WORKSHEET FOR CHAPTER ONE

1. What pain relief techniques have you used in the past?

2. If you are experiencing pain, where are you in the pain spectrum?

acute	persistent	chronic

3. How would you classify your intensity of pain throughout most of the day?

1			10
low	becoming intrusive	very intrusive	severe

CHAPTER TWO

TYPES OF PAIN
AND PAIN RELIEF

The Nature of the Dance

We think of choreography as relating to dance. On the surface of
it, that's a pretty far-out metaphor to describe the experience of
one in pain. However, if we think of some things (people, factors,
situations) as shifting or moving *in relation to* other things (people, factors, situations) then we can certainly apply the concept
of choreography to what happens in the life of a person in pain
as his or her whole life begins to inevitably revolve around that
pain.

This is the origin of the metaphor. But before we begin to explore it, let's look at some more definitions.

DEFINITIONS

DANCE: to move in a rhythmic or stylized way. You can dance
by yourself, with another, or in a group. A dance can be formal
or completely informal, structured or unstructured. There can be
many rhythms to a dance. Above all, for our purposes especially,
we must remember that a dance is an **expression**.

And what, for our purposes here, is the dance expressing? Anger. Suffering. Helplessness.

Let's look further at this metaphor of pain being a dance, and see how it fits in with our various definitions from Chapter One.

Acute Pain

As I have already said, acute pain is a "positive pain." There is a reason for it, easily perceived and understood. It might be intense, but we are reasonably sure that it will be short-lived.

Usually, with acute pain, you are dancing with yourself, either all of yourself or part of yourself. Acute pain can be an extremely dissociative experience. People often describe floating above themselves, seeing the emergency crew working on them as they lie on the roadway, or watching from a distance. They usually report that they did not feel any pain while they were in that dissociated state. Some are able to spontaneously modify or modulate the experience by deliberately modifying the dissociative aspect, whatever it might be—floating higher, or watching from further away. Usually this is not a conscious decision; the subconscious mind knows that such modulation will be helpful. It is particularly likely to happen if the person knows that there is no other immediate pain-relief in sight, because they are still on the ski slope, for example, and they have a dislocated hip. Somehow the subconscious mind flips into its "Great Protector" mode and creates the dissociative experience. In almost all respects, it is similar to an hypnotic experience, and often people who are skilled in self-hypnosis can do this quite deliberately and successfully.

In our metaphor, The Dance of Acute Pain is usually choreographed around a specific event or experience, and The Dance is finished when that experience or event is over—the appendix is out, the person is successfully carried down from the ski slope to the waiting ambulance and subsequently the hip is restored to its socket, the motor vehicle accident is a thing of the past and the injuries are healing. The choreography changes as recovery proceeds—the closing scenes of that particular Dance.

Think of the woman who is having repeated gall bladder attacks. We'll call her Mary. For a while, perhaps, Mary says nothing to her family, thinking that these episodes are due to "a flu bug," or indiscriminate eating, or that they just "are." One evening, however, about an hour and a half after dinner, she begins to experience such acute pain that she doubles over. She can't walk or even sit in a chair. The pain is awful—far worse than anything she has experienced before—and she knows that she is going to have to do something about it.

Up to this point, this has been a little dance (or a series of little dances) with Mary herself, with maybe some bit parts danced by a concerned family member; now, however, those small roles become more prominent as someone calls the doctor and Mary heads off to the emergency room.

For a short scene, other people come on stage—admitting clerks, nurses, lab technicians, the family doctor and the surgeon; nevertheless, Mary does not feel particularly connected to these people. She is too involved in her own pain. She hears the doctors tell her that she has an acute obstruction of the gall bladder and they feel that immediate surgery is indicated, but their voices come from a distance. Something jogs her memory—don't they usually treat gall bladder attacks with some kind of medication?—but then another wave of pain hits her. The supporting cast is far away; she is really dancing a solo.

When she wakes up from the anaesthetic, her abdomen is sore and it's kind of hard to move, but this discomfort is nothing compared to the pre-operative pain. She stays in the hospital for a few days and the other members of the company dance their small roles, but the pain subsides steadily. The Dance is over.

Persistent Pain

When some misfortune occurs and the acute pain experience does not abate—some complication of injury, or the added component of severe psychological stress such as war or natural catastrophe—then the pain may go on and become persistent. Persistent pain can be continual (that is, it is there all the time) or continuous (it is there off and on).

In The Dance of Persistent Pain, there may be more than one principal dancer. One might liken it to an event at a discordant ballet, rather than to a dance routine. There is almost always more outside/inside influence than with acute pain. And The Dance has become intrusive, spilling over into the person's daily life.

This may have happened to the worker we were thinking of in Chapter One. The complicating influences could have been financial stress, a feeling of guilt that the injury had occurred ("If I hadn't been such a klutz, it wouldn't have happened") or worthlessness ("What good am I to my family if I can't even work?") or it could have been some unexpected complication of the injury—it hadn't healed well, or other impairment had been hidden by the more overt problem.

Or perhaps Mary's convalescence did not go well and she continued to have abdominal pain every day. She was confused and angry and she wondered what had gone wrong. Maybe they shouldn't have operated after all. Maybe something happened during the surgery that they didn't tell her about. Maybe she had cancer and they weren't telling her. Other people were becoming more visible on the stage as the pain continued long after she thought she was going to be better.

As this situation continues, the pain sufferer begins to choreograph his or her life around the pain. The rest of the world, so to speak, becomes drawn into The Dance. *This is not an intentional action by the patient.* It is due to the particular confluence of factors in any one case.

Unfortunately, as pain-filled day follows pain-filled day, the pain becomes *chronic*, and the person is developing a "Chronic Pain Syndrome."

Chronic Pain

Chronic pain is a "negative" pain; it seems to have no purpose. There may have *been* a purpose, in earlier days—as protection, perhaps—but no one can find such a reason now. Mary's gall bladder is out. The worker's injuries are theoretically healed. Mary should be cheerfully and comfortably carrying on with her life; the worker should be back at work.

Yet—*and this is the important part*—the pain continues. It is not imaginary; it is real. But no one can answer the question, "Why is this person still having pain?"

The Dance of Chronic Pain begins to, and eventually does, involve many outside dance partners. No longer is this a dance mainly with the self: it becomes a dance with one's immediate world, and everybody and everything in it.

Samantha knew that this couldn't go on forever. It was bizarre that she should have gone into the hospital for three days and still be there weeks—months—later. She was fine as long as she was on heavy medication, but she knew that she couldn't possibly do her job in that drugged state.

Her folks were getting very worried too—her husband, and her parents. She could see the concern on their faces, hear it in their voices as they "tried" to be cheerful. She wished they would just stay away, not come to visit her at all. It made her feel worse than ever and sometimes she felt like yelling at them, "GO HOME! LEAVE ME ALONE!" Then she felt guilty and that gave her something more to feel bad about.

She was again wondering what she was doing wrong, how she was making herself worse. It *had* to be all her fault because she was again getting those vibes from the nurses—as if she was taking up a bed that someone else needed more than she did. ("You're just going to have to change your attitude—learn to live with it. After all, other people get headaches too.")

But not like mine, she thought helplessly. Not like mine.

PAIN RELIEF TECHNIQUES

Let us go back a bit, and talk more now about various ways of relieving pain.

Earlier I suggested that there were basically two types of pain relief techniques: those that applied more directly to the conscious mind, and those that were directed more to the subconscious.

Situations involving acute pain generally rely on those techniques which relieve the physiological aspects of pain. Medication is usually the first one that most people think of (although one could argue the wisdom of that). This may range from the mildest analgesic, such as aspirin or Tylenol, to the heaviest of heavy-duty substances, such as morphine or heroin or some type of anaesthesia, which could be local (as we might get at the dentist's or when having a laceration sutured), or general (as for most surgery).

Medications work by interacting with brain chemistry to reduce pain-producing substances (e.g., substance-P in the central nervous system chemistry) or replace them with comfort-producing substances (e.g., serotonin). This is a pretty simplistic way to portray the complex neurophysiology of pain, but it will do for our purposes here. Usually, with medication, there is a simultaneous increase in one's sense of well-being, partly because the same or very similar biochemistry is involved.

The relief of pain allows the body to relax, and this in turn encourages healing. With healing, pain diminishes and the body no longer needs to express its anger.

Physical techniques such as the application of ice or heat will often relieve acute pain. Sometimes I think that sports teams must just about own the ice-manufacturing industry! Generally, ice will reduce swelling and spasm quite effectively when applied soon after injury, and heat will bring more comfort to the pain of arthritis. (Arthritis is a good example of a chronic *condition* which has acute flare-ups.)

Physical support, from a sling or cast, is another type of pain-relief approach which is particularly applicable to acute situations such as injuries. The question of when to move a painful part of the body and when to protect it from movement is also important for maintaining comfort.

At times, surgical intervention is necessary to relieve pain, because the pain is a clear message that there is something drastically wrong inside our bodies. Gall bladder attacks, appendicitis, or a potential disaster from a ruptured organ are good examples of this. With successful surgery, the pain is relieved, although there still may be some necessity for analgesia to relieve postoperative pain.

Unfortunately, it sometimes happens that surgery is undergone again and again in an attempt to relieve pain which has no clear surgical indication. This is a travesty of medical care, but one can understand why some patients, desperate for relief, and some surgeons, desperate to help their patients find some relief, at times fall into this trap. When the expected results from surgery (or other forms of treatment) have not occurred, a more clear-sighted investigation needs to be done. Rarely is more surgery the answer.

Reassessment of ALL the factors in that person's life is mandatory. This needs to be suggested with great tact and diplomacy; we are all very reluctant to look at some of these issues—those that involve relationships, for instance, or the way we respond to the demands put upon us. Deep down inside, we know that those factors which we are most reluctant to look at are the very ones which need to be explored.

Are there cases where surgeons have gone ahead with less-than-pristine motives? Yes. This is called malpractice. Protect yourself with second opinions. However, when those opinions that have gone before have not been what you want to hear, third and fourth and fifth opinions always compound rather than relieve the situation. A different approach is indicated.

The more psychologically directed approaches play a role in the relief of acute pain. For example, anything that will release and reduce muscle tension, such as relaxation techniques, will bring some relief. This is what happens, of course, when a painful part is supported with a sling or a cast. Again, this is because ALL pain, whatever its origin, has some muscle-tension component. After all, the natural tendency of the body, when there is pain, is to *splint itself* when there is no mechanical splint available—to hold itself *still*, because moving the painful part hurts. Unfortunately this is also an unintentional self-sabotage because a tight, tense muscle is always more uncomfortable than a relaxed muscle. The trick, obviously, is to achieve a relaxed muscle while still preventing much movement.

Distraction is also a useful pain reliever. Most of us do this spontaneously when we have some pain (a headache, for example) but we have to get on with the job at hand. Sometimes we will say, "I just don't have time for this headache right now" and then realize, some time later, that it has gone. The subconscious seems to have a built-in priority evaluator that lets us know what must take precedence. The more desperate the distraction, the more effective it is: think of the mother whose child is in danger—she ignores her pain completely until she knows her child is safe. Similarly, the athlete who is injured in a competition often doesn't even know he's injured until the competition is over.

Children are spectacularly good at distraction and can often endure very painful procedures, such as intravenous punctures, without a flinch if someone is reading them their favorite story.

When we get into the realm of Persistent Pain, the picture begins to change.

Patients will complain that the pills don't work any more, or that there is nothing they can do to get relief. This is a very dangerous interlude in the pain spectrum, because it will lead directly to chronic pain and all that that entails unless it is vigorously attended to while it is still in the 'persistent' stage.

This is not easy. The pain is already intrusive and the patient's natural protective mechanisms are getting into gear. With these, there is the subtle beginning of a shift in attitude—not conscious (*never* conscious, I believe) but potentially very sabotaging.

Think back to our work-related casualty. He or she is definitely at that very dangerous stage. A kind of desperation is setting in. With the desperation comes a monstrous increase in the feelings of helplessness and—always a companion of helplessness—hopelessness.

As the sufferer slides relentlessly into a chronic situation, almost invariably the medication becomes less and less useful. Higher doses definitely do not help. Stronger medications, which may bring relief for a time, do not bring a sustained relief. The risk for 'polypharmacy' is very high as people—both patients and doctors—search for other and/or more effective medications. After a while, the patient may be taking far too many pills, all at the same time, with the consequent possibility of drug interaction or sensitivity. Some drugs stay in the system for a longer time than others, too, which means further risks of building up blood levels of some medication to toxic levels. This is a potentially dangerous situation, both medically and psychologically, as the patient becomes more and more desperate to find relief. We could say that complications are too close for comfort—literally.

I believe this is the stage when approaches should be directed more toward the subconscious mind, rather than just toward the cognitive, intellectualizing mind or physical body.

Suffering is emotional. We *feel* it, far more than just physically. It has nothing to do with logic. Why, then, should we think that we can ignore attending to the needs of the subconscious—the part of the brain where emotions are processed?

One of the first hurdles is helping the sufferer to understand that these techniques are active interventions for the relief of the *suffering* component of pain. The sufferer needs to be reassured, often many times over, that—for reasons which we simply do not understand—the conventional, physiologically-directed pain relief techniques are not very useful now, and that leaves us with the challenge of assisting him or her in finding strengths and resources from within, to ease the *distress* of pain, the intrusion of pain, into every moment of that person's life. The pain sufferer must be released from the implication that the pain is "all the patient's fault." Patients will often relate that they have pain even when they are asleep. I believe them.

Subconsciously-directed techniques will be described in more detail, with examples, in Chapter Six, but I will give a little rundown here.

"Relaxation" is a word that sets off jangling bells in the minds of many people. The connotation is of some airy-fairy state of bliss—hardly a suggestion that would be taken kindly by a chronic pain patient.

It is more useful, and certainly more accurate, to speak of "the release of muscle tension." *That* is a concept that can be understood by anyone in pain, because the tension throughout the body is extremely high. As I mentioned before, the natural tendency of the body when there is pain is to splint the pain by holding the affected part tight and, obviously, tense. Unfortunately, although the prevention of movement has a useful effect in the short term, tightness and tension usually over-ride it, and pain is exacerbated rather than relieved.

Initially, people often have a hard time believing this. One way to demonstrate it is to ask the person to deliberately make the painful part (or ANY part) of the body even tighter: tighter and tighter and more and more tense, and tighter and tighter and more and more tense, and then—whoof! Let the tightness suddenly go. The relief will be immediate.

We need to shift the definition of "relaxation" to mean "the release of muscle tension" so that it makes more sense—and is more easily accepted.

"Dissociation" is the experience of putting either some distance, or a barrier, between oneself and what is going on. The most common reason to use dissociation to ease pain is to put some distance between oneself and one's pain. We saw earlier that many people do this spontaneously during traumatic events. Sometimes people do it so successfully that they develop an amnesia barrier—they don't remember what happened. This is not uncommon with motor vehicle accidents, or other kinds of trauma (including emotional trauma). Usually the amnesia breaks down as time goes on, injuries heal and the subconscious begins to feed information back to the conscious mind. But many experience that rather strange "watching-from-above" phenomenon and can describe the situation in exact and intricate detail later. The dissociation has protected the injured person from experiencing pain during those minutes or hours. When they are safe again, the sensation of pain returns. By then, it is hoped, the injuries have been attended to and are healing or, if there is pain, it is of the acute variety that people recognize as being appropriate in the circumstances—a "positive" pain.

Sometimes, when a person has been badly injured and he or she has been in a coma for some period of time, the increasing awareness of pain as that person comes out of the coma is one of the body's ways of telling the victim that s/he is alive.

Distraction is very similar to dissociation but is often a more deliberate separation. As I mentioned before, children are positively gifted at doing this; people who work with children who have cancer have found that many of the painful procedures which the children have to go through in the course of their therapy are easily ignored by the child when someone (preferably someone special—a parent or special friend) engages the child's imagination in some way—a story, pop-up-books, asking questions such as "how many things can you think of that are green?" and similar games.

When adults use distraction it is often more mundane (which is too bad, I often think!). Sarah has a term paper which must be in tomorrow and she resolutely puts the pain in her back, which she incurred falling off her bike, further away from her awareness than the task at hand. Or one might involve oneself in one's favorite hobby, or ask a friend over for tea. These techniques work well for the acute pain situation and they are also useful for easing chronic pain. The extent of the relief often depends on the willingness of the patient to explore these possibilities. That's all very well to say, but not so easy to do when one is already in the vicious cycle of pain–fear–pain. One suggestion that seems sensible is to experiment at whatever time of day one has found to be the least infused with pain. For some, this might be when they just get up after a night's sleep; for others, the times when there is some relief from medication might be appropriate.

Those of you who are reading this book because you are in a pain cycle of your own will know what I mean, and will also know how hard it is to wrest oneself from the depths of the helpless/hopeless vortex. It just makes sense to use whatever advantage one can find.

Remember also that *pain itself* is a dissociative experience, as we discussed in Chapter One, and we can tap into that ready-made framework when we are looking at these possibilities.

The biggest group of pain relief approaches that invoke the subconscious, more than the conscious mind, are those which have the ability to bring about an altered state of consciousness—meditation, yoga, hypnosis, and autogenic training. When we are in such an altered state, the muscles in the body release some of their tension (we've already talked about the advantages of that), and create some distance between oneself and one's pain because of the involvement with the altered state.

There is another altered state that is very important for some people, and that is the state of deep prayer. I'm not talking about the shriek of "Oh, God, help me!"—as crucial as that is in some situations. I mean the intense involvement between one's spirit and a personal Higher Power, whatever one wants to call it, that lifts one away from the chaotic world into a place of peace.

Biofeedback also utilizes an intense concentration (which is a type of altered state) combined with instrumentation that gives the person evidence of something happening—a pulse, a temperature change, etc. It's nice to have some corroboration! One then focuses on creating the internal environment which brings about the desired change. One of the best examples of this is the use of biofeedback to relieve migraines by diverting the blood-flow away from the cranial arteries toward the hands, thus warming the hands. The focus is on experiencing the hands getting warmer, which happens, thus directing more blood to the hands than to the head. Because migraines have to do with the diameter and dilatation of the cranial blood vessels, reducing the blood flow allows for a shrinkage in diameter of those small arteries. Arteries whose walls are on the stretch are very painful. As there are thousands of microscopic nerve endings in the arterial walls, when the stretch eases, so does the pain. Conversely, spasm can be excruciatingly painful, too, as anyone who has ever had a cramp can attest.

Biofeedback bridges the conscious and subconscious techniques; so do acupuncture and acupressure. These latter skills are not in my repertoire, so I cannot speak knowledgeably about them, except to say that they are very, very useful in some cases and are worth investigating.

Although we have drifted somewhat away from our metaphor of The Dance, we have just been setting the scene. In the following chapters, we will find out more about The Dance and how it can help in relieving chronic pain.

Samantha was eventually discharged from the hospital but it seemed not so much to be that a magic combination of medication had been found, as it was that she had come through some kind of cycle which finally just wound down.

Nevertheless, she was still on a lot of medication and her neurologist had told her in no uncertain terms that she should take time off from work.

"How much time?" she asked, thinking in terms of a few weeks and mentally organizing her projects around that.

"One year."

"One YEAR? That's impossible! I can't leave my work for one YEAR! How would I ever catch up again? Even if someone took over the projects, after a year I'd be so out of touch—"

"One year."

Feeling desperate, she talked it over with her husband, Dave. She thought that he would support her side but he had a different viewpoint and thought that one year off was a good idea. Financially they could manage—they'd have to watch their spending a bit but they were lucky enough to be able to get along without her income.

Hardly able to comprehend what was happening to her, she arranged the leave of absence. Then she discovered that Dave and her parents had another bomb to throw at her. They wanted her to go to see a doctor who did hypnosis.

The only reason she agreed was to get them off her back.

PERTINENT POINTS FROM CHAPTER TWO

The **choreography** we are describing refers to people, factors, and situations shifting or moving **in relation** to other people, factors, or situations.

"Dance" is an **expression**—the dance of pain expresses anger, suffering, helplessness, and hopelessness.

Acute pain has a purpose and usually lasts a limited time; **persistent** pain extends past the time when relief and/or recovery would have been expected; **chronic** pain continues long after any 'reason' for the pain can be found.

There is a variety of pain-relief techniques, some of which are directed to the conscious mind, and some more to the subconscious mind.

With chronic pain syndromes, it is important to explore those techniques which engage the **subconscious mind.**

WORKSHEET FOR CHAPTER TWO

1. How do I define The Dance and the dancers in my situation?

2. Where do I fit into this scene?

3. For how long have I been part of this Dance?

4. Has The Dance changed from what it was in the beginning?

   When?

   How?

CHAPTER THREE

THE ROLE OF PAIN IN YOUR LIFE

The Purpose of the Dance

What role does pain play in our lives?

For those of us who are lucky enough to be pain-free most of the time, pain plays a very minor role indeed. For many of us, ageing brings on aches and pains having to do with wear and tear on the body, and such conditions as osteoporosis, early arthritides of one sort or another, the dull ache of soft tissue rheumatism, or muscles unused to strenuous exercise that complain after we shovel the snow off the driveway. These are annoying, relatively minor problems—more or less transient in nature.

But for people who have some sort of chronic painful condition, the pain itself has a leading role in day-to-day living. What good does that do, we wonder? Why are we thus afflicted? What's the *purpose* of pain?

Or, to continue with the metaphor, what is the purpose of The Dance?

COMMUNICATION

The Dance of pain has one purpose: communication.

This could be communication with the self, to warn of a problem developing, or communication with the family or close associates, or communication with the larger community, such as the medical or legal community.

Acute pain, as we saw in Chapter Two, is usually a communication with the self, to warn of something happening that shouldn't be happening in the body. The pain sufferer may then go on to describe the pain to someone else—a doctor or a friend or relative—so that is a secondary communication, but it is directly related to the first: a warning and a quest for help.

Let's go back to Mary, with her gall bladder attack. First, her body was sending a communication to *her*: "Something is really awry here, Mary, and you're going to have to do something about it." Because Mary had ignored the earlier warnings, when surgery might have been avoided (remember, she didn't know that at the time, and retrospective vision is always 20/20) her body finally sent a message much louder and clearer, demanding action. This communication then was sent out from Mary to her family, who contacted the doctor, and action did in fact proceed from there.

Injuries are usually painful, and the message here is often one of admonition: "Be more careful!" The discomfort is also a way to ensure that further damage does not take place, because one naturally protects the vulnerable injured part.

The pain of angina is a sharp warning, literally, from the heart: "Hey! I'm not getting enough oxygen! Slow down, or take your nitro, or follow whatever other instructions your doctor has given you!"

These warnings are for protection—the mind and body are communicating well and telling each other what each needs to know in order to protect the health of the body. The communication as it is *sent*, is excellent, but remember that communication involves a receiver, too. We also have to *respond* appropriately.

So when 62-year-old Joe experiences pain in his chest while shoveling the snow from the driveway, the communication is clear: "Something is wrong here—stop shovelling and find out what is happening." The communication is also a statement, to oneself and to others. In acute pain, the statement from within is: "I want you to pay attention to me. This is important."

When pain becomes persistent, the communication gradually assumes a different character. What was a warning in the acute pain situation becomes a cry for help in the persistent situation. There is still the need for protection, but it is more to prevent one from sliding into the chronic scenario than from some disaster occurring in the body. And the statement to the self becomes: "You've got to DO something about this! It's getting out of hand!" That same statement is subsequently directed to others, especially the medical community: "DO something! PLEASE!!"

"Post-whiplash syndrome" often fits into this category, as do other injuries which apparently heal, but the injured person still experiences pain. The situation becomes more and more stressful, thus intensifying the pain. There may be overt as well as covert anger, which of course adds more tension and stress. The injured person may seem hard to get along with, because of his or her frustration that the problem isn't going away, so family members are drawn into The Dance and they have their ways of communicating, also. In a different way, friends and relatives express their frustration, and may add their voices to the victim's: "Why doesn't somebody DO something?"

Pain is generally classified as 'chronic' when it has gone on for six months or more. Usually the original instigating factors, such as an injury, have—as far as anyone can determine—healed. Yet the pain persists and by now it is intruding so intensely into the sufferer's life that it begins to take over. No longer is the primary purpose of communication one of warning or even protection. The new statement becomes a way of expressing the anger. It is the means of saying, to the world and to the self: "I AM SUF-FERING!"

This is probably as good a time as any to talk about a term that offends many people. The term is "secondary gain." It is a term which is heard frequently on rehabilitation units, in chronic disorders programs, in pain clinics, by doctors, nurses, psychologists, physiotherapists, lawyers, and claims adjusters. But from the sufferer's perspective—"Whoa! What do you mean, "secondary GAIN? *What* gain?"

Well, let's talk about a few possibilities—and the first thing to say is, we are not talking about malingering, which is a deliberate intent to deceive. We are talking about perfectly normal, understandable psychological processes that evolve in almost all chronic situations. How could anybody experience pain for six

months or more and not have an emotional or psychological reaction to that? It wouldn't make sense.

How often has a victim of a motor vehicle accident experienced
increasing pain as the wheels of the judiciary and legal systems
grind on—and on—and on. Then, when the case is finally settled,
after a while the pain begins to subside. Has the person been deliberately deceiving everybody about the nature of his injuries and
the intensity of his pain? Of course not. What has happened is
that the increasing stress of the lengthy legal proceedings has been
the culprit. Of course stress exacerbates pain. Such exacerbation
occurs through many routes—one of the most obvious is plain
old-fashioned tension. Tension fosters tight muscles. Tight, tense
muscles are in themselves more painful than relaxed muscles. (We
can, and have, and will say this over and over again!) When the
whole affair has finally come to an end, the tension begins to ebb
away and so does some of the pain.

Here is another common scenario.

Let us imagine a family in which relationships are under
quite a strain. There are no overt nasty things happening
but no one is very happy. Suddenly Joan, the mother, is
rear-ended when she is sitting innocently at a red light.
She sustains a severe whiplash injury. Her car is badly
damaged—it was quite a crash. She has no other notable
injuries except the abrasion from her seat belt as it held
her safely against the force of the collision.

Suddenly Joan's family has a new focus. They are all
concerned about Joan. People seem to be getting along better, and everyone is very solicitous of her. She is in quite
severe pain for days and days and then it becomes sort
of a boring ache that is, in many ways, even harder to
put up with. She goes dutifully to physiotherapy but it
doesn't help much. Her doctor gives her a variety of medications to relieve pain, reduce spasm, and soothe her nerves.

"Post-whiplash syndrome" is a real entity, well-
documented. It can go on for a long time with sleep disturbances, trouble concentrating, a feeling as if the head
isn't quite connected to the shoulders properly, pain and
spasm in the neck and perhaps in the back, feelings of anxiety and a general lack of well-being.

Months go by. The acute worry about Joan is over, and is replaced by a new one: "Why isn't she getting better? Is something else wrong?" So once again the family has a new focus, and once again some of the just-under-the-surface abrasions are pushed further down. Joan is relying heavily on her husband, and that is a new experience for him. He responds with even more solicitude.

Joan is not deliberately playing any games here. She is truly suffering. One of the few 'positive' things about the whole situation—and one of the 'gains' to Joan—is the more comfortable relationship within the family. That is what is known as 'secondary gain.' It happens subconsciously. It is a normal, human response.

TYPES OF COMMUNICATION

So far I have been talking about the messages that pain communicates from within a person to that person him/herself, to the family and immediate contacts, and to the wider community.

How is that pain *expressed* in these communications? And how are these messages perceived?

"Communication" means far more than verbal exchange. Often the *way* we use words, more than the words themselves, sends the stronger message; and there are always other clues, such as visual clues, which are important factors.

There is usually not much question about the message of acute pain. The words, the posture, the obvious effort required of the person to speak through intense pain make it clear. And its message is perceived clearly, also—seldom does someone question the patient who comes in to the emergency ward doubled over, staggering a little in the effort to walk, saying through gritted teeth, "I have a terrible pain in my lower back—I was just bending over to move a small chair and when I tried to straighten up I nearly fainted with the pain—just like a vise—it's terrible, terrible." The person's face is contorted, and he or she may be ashen as the autonomic nervous system responds to the pain.

This poor individual probably has acute lumbosacral spasm and is in desperate need of some medication. Lucky are the souls who can do relaxation techniques or self-hypnosis to get through such an episode! Most can't—the pain came out of the blue; there was no time for preparation. One was in the throes of it before he or she even had a chance to recognize what was happening. Once the spasm has been broken by medication, however, and there is a chance to breathe and even (*very* gingerly) move again, such techniques might be used effectively.

If pain becomes persistent, the communication begins to change—in both directions. The tone of voice changes—is anyone out there *listening?*—and becomes more insistent. This tone is recognized immediately by whomever is receiving this communication, and that person's response is colored by his or her frustration, and this is obvious to the patient. The listener's response may come across as anger or dismissal, neither of which sits very well with the person in pain. It may also inspire the beginnings of guilt: "I'm doing all I can but nothing is working, so I mustn't be doing enough."

Let's say that Sam had a freak accident at work—a shelf gave way and some equipment caught his elbow as it crashed to the floor. There was no question of it being his fault; the real culprit was whoever had put the shelf up in that spot in the first place, but that person probably was long gone and nobody would remember who it was anyway.

Sam received workers' compensation and took three weeks off work because the doctor had said that there was very deep bruising and probably even some bleeding under the periosteum (the membranous covering of the bone). That should have been that, but for some reason the healing process didn't proceed as was expected and, after a month, Sam still wasn't back at work because he couldn't bend his elbow without pain.

After the sixth week, he phoned his boss to say that he still couldn't return to work. The boss received this news with a marked lack of enthusiasm. Sam was a valuable employee and it was hard to find someone to take over all his tasks.

"It still hurts, does it?" asked the boss.

(Of course it still hurts, you idiot, why do you think I'm phoning?) "Yeah, I'm in quite a lot of pain most of the time and if I try to lift something—forget it."

"Um. Well. . . . (long pause, during which Sam became increasingly fidgety) I guess you're going to have to stay off longer then. But you'll get back as soon as you can, won't you? We don't have very many extra hands around here and there's a flu going around, too." (THAT'S NOT MY FAULT, thinks Sam.)

This exchange does not do much for Sam *or* his boss, and the underlying messages implied in the words and tone of voice come through loud and clear. Sam feels increasingly misunderstood; the boss feels increasingly irritated. On top of all that, there may be the niggling stirrings of guilt in Sam—maybe he should have moved faster—and therefore some defensiveness, which makes him feel even worse.

In the chronic scenario, the whole problem of communication escalates and becomes more and more convoluted. By now the patient is perceived as having developed a 'pain persona.' Such patients may be perceived as exaggerating their symptoms, and comments about 'secondary gain' begin appearing on their charts. His or her reception in the doctor's office or emergency room is cool, to say the least—a communication implied far more through facial expression, tone of voice, and posture than through words. The patient may feel as if everybody is getting fed up with him or her, and that's not far off the mark.

(It's nothing, though, compared to how fed up they are getting with themselves.)

The risk of communication breakdown is high; misinterpretations abound.

Many years ago, I used to do a regular session at a long-term care facility in Vancouver, offering hypnosis and/or counselling to any patients who might benefit from it.

One day I received a referral from one of the doctors to see a young man who had had a terrible motorcycle accident and had sustained a fracture-dislocation very high up in the cervical spine (C2–3). He had become quadriplegic, and had no sensation or movement below the neck. His brain, though, was intact and there was nothing wrong with his intellect.

This young man was driving everybody crazy, complaining that he had a full rectum. He would call the nurses several times a day, saying that stool needed to be evacuated, that he was in pain from the pressure. In fact, (a) seldom was there stool in the rectum, and (b) because he was paralyzed, obviously he had no sensation in that part of his body so why would he complain about how it "felt"?*

I went to see him. He was such an angry young man—in his early twenties, and living a life now destined to be spent in a hospital bed.

We had a long talk. I had a suspicion about what he was *really* wanting to communicate, and after some further discussion I offered a suggestion that might allow him his needs and yet help the nursing staff by lowering the demands. He agreed.

When I went back to the nursing station, I had another long talk, this time with the nurses, and I finished by saying, "If the only way you knew that you were alive below the neck was to feel as if your rectum was uncomfortably full, wouldn't you want to keep that sensation?"

THIS was the real communication, and they understood. My suggestion to the patient was that he and the nurses agree on a contract: they would check for stool twice a day, without fail, and he would therefore not have to call them for that service.

All parties agreed, and the "problem" (one very small part of this young man's total problem) was solved.

Those of us who are therapists need to remember that it is always worthwhile, with chronic pain patients, to take time to straighten out any communication barriers. By the time the patient has advanced to chronic pain status, there are huge overlayers of communication. These are not easily dealt with and must be discussed with tact and candor (no small feat!). "Listen with the third ear"—to adapt a psychotherapy phrase. We must use *all* our senses—visual, auditory, postural, verbal, and a good dollop of ESP—to help our patients and clients communicate their real needs.

---

*Although this long-held belief may be refuted in light of some recent research (see the work of Melzack and of Katz in the "Research and Literature" section), I don't think the newer theories interfere with the validity of taking a different approach.

Body language—theirs and ours; facial expression—ditto; the actual words with which we phrase our thoughts and questions and, of course, tone of voice. And we need to ask simple questions: "What is it that is troubling you most *right now*?"

With such empathic attention, communication in both directions improves tremendously. And of course, remember about the anger and guilt in both patient and caregivers—for the caregivers because nothing they do is helping; for the patient because what is being done is not helping—"What's wrong with me?"

We often underestimate the impact of our communications. That's because we pay more attention to the conscious, cognitive functions of the brain than to its unconscious, experiential functions. How many physicians remember to write a prescription thus: "Take two tablets every six hours as required for the *relief* of pain" rather than thus: "Take two tablets every six hours for pain." Do we *really* want our patients to have pain every six hours?

Or this well-known piece of advice: "You're just going to have to learn to live with it." (Corollary: Without it, will I die?)

Now, it is unrealistic to have to stop and examine every word before we say it, check our body posture and language, compose our faces, etc., etc., etc. But we *can* pay close attention to what our patients are telling us, and HOW they are telling us those things. Re-framing a comment is a great psychotherapy technique, and it can clarify murky messages wonderfully well.

PATIENT: I'm afraid that my wife won't be able to cope much longer.
THERAPIST: Let me just make sure of what you mean by that. Could you say a little more about it?
PATIENT: Well, she's getting pretty worn out—taking care of me and all—
THERAPIST: It sounds as if you may be feeling that you're a burden on her.
PATIENT: Well, I AM, aren't I? I can't work, can't take care of myself—she has to drive me everywhere—
THERAPIST: Is there another way that we could phrase your concern, to clarify it?
PATIENT: (Squirming a little, obviously unhappy): Well. . . .

THERAPIST: (Gently, but firmly): Are you afraid she might leave you?
PATIENT: (Blurting it out): Well, she might, mightn't she? I mean, there's nothing for her to stay for—a good woman like that deserves better than having to take care of a cripple all the time!
THERAPIST: Maybe she would have a different perspective on that. Let's talk a little bit more about what has brought these worries into your mind.

Now that they have come to the true crux of the matter, the patient's anxieties can be brought to the surface and his terror of being left can be discussed, perhaps with the wife present and included in the discussion.

Here's an entirely different Dance scene.

Let's say that you had been involved in a dreadful accident. A family member had been killed, and although you were badly hurt, you tried your best to help him or her.

Over the ensuing months, your pain worsened although the injuries were apparently healing as well as could be expected. At first this exasperated you, then frustrated you, then began to anger you.

You also became more and more convinced that you could have done *something* more to help your relative, and when friends and family did their best to reassure you, you became angry both at them and at yourself. Consequently you began to feel guilty about inflicting your anger on those around you and this began to turn into a spiral of pain-guilt-anger-pain-guilt-anger.

This would be a good time to talk to a therapist or counselor, who could help you to forgive yourself and realize that pain makes ogres of us all.

Samantha was a clear historian, describing her situation in a straightforward way; a little *too* straightforward, I thought—she has had to tell this many times over. I wonder how much she expects to be believed?

There was little hesitation in responding to my question about how the pain intruded into her life. "I can't do my work. If I'm in pain, the pain interferes with my ability to think clearly. If I take the medication, I'm too befuddled with the drugs.

"And I never know if I am going to be able to keep a luncheon engagement, or visit friends or have them over . . ."

"And your husband?" I asked.

"He's wonderful—my greatest strength and support. He *accepts* me the way I am. He's one of the very few who do— or can."

"And your love life?" I asked gently.

Her eyes slowly filled with tears as she looked at me: "Hardly ever, any more."

We began to talk about practicalities—what we might reasonably hope she might achieve by learning hypnotic techniques, the frequency of appointments, cost, and all those mundane but necessary things. She was a bit more relaxed than when she had first come in, and obviously had decided that she was willing to find out a little bit more about some new approaches. We set up an introductory series of appointments.

Communication can be verbal or nonverbal, overt or covert, conscious or subconscious, simple or complex, literal or figurative, intellectual or emotional. Often we slip into the conscious, overt, simple, verbal, literal intellectual mode because it feels safe—there's not much room for **feelings**. Feelings can be too scary. But until we as clinicians help explore the feelings, and put them into context, we are not fulfilling our task for our patients. And until we as patients can begin such an exploration, we are shielding our real selves. When we are dealing with something as complex as pain, especially long-lasting pain, our feelings are the source of many truths. Take that leap into the unknown and find out where your deepest fears—and your deepest strengths—are hiding.

Pain is the communicating link.

Before closing off this chapter, I want to talk about the communication involved in phantom limb pain, and also in the pain associated with diseases like irritable bowel syndrome and fibromyalgia.

There are some chronic pain syndromes which seem to be more closely linked with what are called "body memories," than are other types of chronic pain.

Phantom limb pain has been known for a long time, of course. It is very common for a patient who has had to have an amputation to suffer excruciating pain in what seems to him to be the amputated limb.

For decades, there seemed to be little reason behind this phenomenon, which was notoriously difficult to treat. Analgesics just didn't touch it. There was some limited success with hypnosis and similar approaches, but 'limited' is the word.

In 1992 and 1993, two papers were published in eminent journals by Dr. J. Katz, which are reviewed in the "Research and Literature" section at the end of the book. In essence, they describe the strong probability of somatosensory memory tracts. In other words, the body remembers, and especially that the body remembers pain.

This work has immense relevance to other disorders which have come into the category of "body memories." The implication is that the body is 'remembering' early painful experiences, which leads us, of course, into the thorny area of child abuse. A higher, statistically significant percentage of adults who suffered extremely abusive childhoods—not only physical or sexual abuse but also emotional abuse—suffer from this type of pain than do people in the unaffected population. In Catchlove's work (see Research and Literature, Chapter Nine), we see that he has found many chronic pain patients to be alexithymic—that is, they have trouble finding words to express their emotions. This also fits the picture: what the brain cannot say, the body may express. With one communication avenue closed, the mind, in its infinite ingenuity, finds another.

Almost all authors who have published on fibromyalgia refer both to the very real physiological abnormalities, such as the distorted serotonin metabolism, and to the psychological correlates. Severely interrupted sleep patterns, with the concomitant alteration in both biochemistry and emotional well-being, is always mentioned, as is poor family communication and sexual dysfunction. Almost all also mention the incidence of co-morbidity with such diagnoses as irritable bowel, irritable bladder, and headache. (Put this into body language: it says volumes about the way the patient thinks of the world—and what she'd like to do to express it.)

Applying the choreography metaphor to these conditions is very easy—they practically beg for such an exploration.

An extremely attractive patient, 46-year-old Mrs. L. M., came originally with chronic pain attributed to an old back injury. In the course of our work together, the focus of the pain shifted to a generalized body pain, which fit the diagnostic parameters of fibromyalgia. She was on a disability pension which required regular re-evaluations (she had ALL the emotional difficulty which is so often associated with that), and she felt strongly that her G.P., for whom she had a high regard, was getting absolutely fed up with her. I know her G.P. and he was not fed up, but he *was* getting very frustrated.

So was I.

I began to ask her, again, what her life was like, how the break-up of her marriage had affected her (we had already talked about it but it bore revisiting), how she was getting along now with her adult son. Without too much difficulty, this led to what she remembered of her childhood.

Well, she remembered quite a lot—especially about needing to be perfect and never quite making it (although by anybody else's standard, she 'made it' in spades). She now lived a long way—a continent and an ocean away—from her childhood home and she had little desire to go back.

Mrs. L. M. does not have huge memory gaps in her recollections. Indeed, she remembers all too clearly. She does not have a history of physical or sexual abuse. On the contrary, nobody even hugged her. But she cringes down inside herself when she thinks of her emotionally sterile formative years and what they did to her ability to express *her* emotions, especially anger.

The alternative communication pathway is pretty clear. Instead of being able to express her emotions verbally or through physical contact—touch, hugs—she diverted it into pain. Together we've been working hard on new ways of communicating, of expressing in words what was so inexpressible for so long. She still has a great deal of pain. But she understands more about where it came from: the choreography of The Dance is changing.

PERTINENT POINTS FROM CHAPTER THREE

The role of pain—the purpose of The Dance—is **communication.**

The message varies depending on the type of pain one experiences: for acute pain, the message is **help;** for persistent pain, **do something;** and for chronic pain, **I am suffering.**

Language is extremely important and we need to pay attention to what we say and how we say it, as well as to what others are saying and how they are saying it.

Some kinds of pain can be identified as **body memories.**

WORKSHEET FOR CHAPTER THREE

1. What am I needing to communicate (there may be more than one thing)?

2. To whom (specifically)?

3. Has my communication broken down in some way?

4. With whom?

5. Just HOW has my communication broken down?

6. Do I know why? (This question is only useful if one includes breakdown in communication with oneself in the *why?*)

7. Are my emotions getting in the way of clear communication?

CHAPTER FOUR

IDENTIFYING YOUR PAIN TRIGGERS

Who Is the Company? Dancers, Directors, and Choreographers

In this chapter we're going to begin to explore the various roles that people may have in this "Dance of Chronic Pain."

From this company, we'll think about the dancers, the director(s) and the choreographer(s). As we do that, the way in which this metaphor reflects the plight of the chronic pain sufferer will become clearer.

First of all, we can consider those who have some attachment to the person in any of several different ways. These will include family, of course, and friends, neighbors, and acquaintances. Fellow workers may very well be involved—and very likely the boss, too.

Then there are the people who are in some way responsible for the medical and/or legal situations in which our sufferer may be involved. These will include doctors and nurses, physio- and occupational therapists, pharmacist and drug store personnel, perhaps (for some) the chiropractor, naturopath or herbalist—maybe even the hypnotherapist! There may also be counselors, psychologists or other psychotherapists. The minister, rabbi or priest may have a very important role. Then there are the people from the various insurance companies or Workers' Compensation boards. Unfortunately there may also be lawyers and judges on the dance stage at times.

Quite a troupe! And those are just the people on the *outside*.

INSIDE DANCERS: EGO STATES AND THEIR ROLES

Everybody has various aspects of his or her personality that are more prominent in one situation or another. I'm a slightly different person when I'm in my office than I am at home, different as a wife than as a mother, different as a friend than as a casual acquaintance. We bring to these various roles/arenas the learning, experience and talents that are connected with whatever it is that we are doing. This is the natural course of events. Such aspects of our personalities are known as "ego states."

We develop such ego states when and how they are needed, and they play a greater or lesser role depending on the circumstances. Sometimes a particular ego state may be prominent for a while, then it subsides back into the subconscious again—the ego state of student or apprentice is a good example. Once the coursework is finished, the exams passed, the certificate bestowed, that particular ego state is not needed, at least for a while.

It is not hard to understand, then, that a similar thing happens when one is ill or in pain for a long time. Such a person develops ego states which help him or her through the days and nights of distress, confusion, anger, grief, and desperation.

These ego states are the "inside dancers" in our metaphor. Often they reflect the various demands which come from the outside members of the company—those whom I have already identified as the various medical and legal professionals who are involved in a patient's life, and upon whom that patient depends so much.

Samantha and I had been working along well for several weeks. She had been a willing subject and quickly learned the basic techniques of relaxation, self-hypnosis, problem-solving and some aspects of hypnotic pain relief. But nothing much was changing in the overall situation—she was still completely incapacitated when the headaches struck, and the pain/fear/pain/fear cycle was as prominent as ever. Late one afternoon we were just finishing up and we talked about what she perceived to be her lack of progress. Without thinking very much about it, I went and xeroxed the overheads which I use when I'm teaching this "choreography" metaphor to my professional colleagues.

"Here," I said as I handed them to her, "take these home and read them over. When you come next time, you can tell me what your thoughts are, and whether you think this approach might be helpful for you."

Over the intervening days I wondered if I had been very wise. Certainly I had never offered the idea in such a way to any other patient—usually I took time to explain the approach carefully and with as much tact as I could muster. Well, we would see if my intuition had played me true or false.

When she came back the next week, she had the xeroxed pages in her hand. "Well?" I asked. "What do you think?"

Rather than answer directly, she told me that her mother was on a trip to Europe for two weeks.

"Oh yes?" I replied, wondering what that had to do with anything.

"She phones me every day, to see if I've got a headache." She paused for a moment. Then—"She's one of the dancers, isn't she?"

"Yes," I said, "she is."

APPLYING THE CONCEPT

Let's think about some examples of chronic pain situations which may make the concept a little clearer.

> Suppose we have a hypothetical patient, Marie. Marie is a teacher, and she has always loved her job. She teaches the younger children, grades two and three. She adores their zest for learning and their wide-eyed acceptance of the world as it is unfolding for them.
>
> When she was a teenager, Marie used to do gymnastics,

and she was quite good at it, usually winning at least some ribbon in any competition she entered.

One day, she made a bad landing on the trampoline. She remembers a sharp pain in her lower back and she was furious with herself for being "such a stupid klutz." She was unable to finish in the competition and therefore missed getting a medal as an all-round athlete of the year.

Her back got better and the pain left, but somehow she never really got back into gymnastics again. She knew that some people said that she was scared. She didn't bother to argue with them. Anyhow, from time to time she *would* get a twitch of that awful pain again, and deep down she thought that maybe being scared was closer to the truth than she wanted to admit.

She remained active in other sports, however—loved skiing and hiking and water sports, and she joined the Outdoor Club when she went to college.

Marie had lots of friends, male and female, and eventually met the man with whom she wanted to spend the rest of her life. They were married when she was twenty-eight and he was thirty, and because they were both strong individualists, there were some stormy times; but they were sincerely committed to each other and to their relationship and worked through the rough spots. On their seventh anniversary, they went out for a gala dinner.

On the way home, they were broadsided by a drunk driver who ran a red light.

Marie's husband, Tim, had a nasty head injury requiring immediate surgery. She paced back and forth in the waiting room for three hours. At long last the neurosurgeon came out and said that Tim was as stable as could be expected, and would be in Intensive Care for an unknown length of time. She could see him, but he was still comatose and wouldn't know her.

Tim recovered, and as he did, a strange thing started to happen to Marie. Her back began hurting, at first just a little niggling discomfort, but it kept getting worse and worse. She went to her doctor, who told her it was nothing to worry about. Probably just stress—and the letdown, now that Tim was out of danger.

The accident had happened in the spring, and during the summer Marie spent a lot of time swimming. It seemed to bring some comfort. However, one day when she and Tim went on a short hike, she had to stop after about half an hour.

"What's wrong?" asked Tim.

"I don't know—my back is really bothering me. I think I'm going to have to go back. I'm sorry to ruin the hike—"

"That's okay," said Tim. But it wasn't, really, thought Marie.

As the summer wore on, she found that all the things that she and Tim loved doing were becoming harder and harder for her. And school was getting closer, too—she would have to start thinking about getting back to work. Somehow, the thought didn't fill her with her usual enthusiasm.

Early in October, Marie went back to her doctor. "My back's killing me," she said. "What on earth is wrong? *Something* must be!" Her doctor examined her and muttered to himself about her range of movement being diminished in both flexion and extension and she seemed to be developing a pelvic tilt. She didn't understand a word of what he was saying—in fact, if the truth be told, she hardly heard him—but when he suggested she see an orthopedic specialist she brightened up. Surely the specialist would find out what was wrong.

Weeks of x-rays, CAT scans, blood tests (*"Blood tests???* It's my BACK!!") and even a muscle biopsy ensued. And the result of all that investigation? "Probably you did more damage than you realized when you had that trampoline accident," the specialist told her, "and the car accident made it flare up again."

"But when will it start getting better? It seems to be worse every day."

"I'll give you some anti-inflammatory medication. That should ease it for you."

"But when?"

"Just start on the medication. I'm sure it will help."

Well, the long and the short of it was that it *didn't* help. The pain still seemed to get worse every day. When she got home after school, all she wanted to do was lie down. At first Tim was very solicitous, brought her a cup of decaf coffee, plumped the pillows up for her, asked her if she wanted anything to read, cooked supper for them (which she seldom wanted but she made herself eat) and gave her a back rub before he kissed her good-night. The back rub *was* wonderful. She always wished it would go on twice as long, but she knew that Tim wanted to get back to his workshop—he was building a model boat.

In time, however, all these ministrations began to pall on Tim. It wasn't that he was deliberately uncaring, but he also couldn't understand what the matter was. And when he approached her sexually, he could feel her tension before he even laid his hand on her. It didn't make for great romance.

Somehow she struggled through the school year. When the end of June came, she knew that, unless there was some major turn-around, she couldn't do it again the next year. The kids needed so *much* of her, and she was short-changing them. It wasn't fair to them, and physically she knew that she just couldn't cope.

Repeated visits to her doctor, to another specialist for a second opinion, and then a third, brought nothing new. Tim was almost like a pleasant stranger. Depression loomed, and her doctor prescribed yet more medication to counteract it. She couldn't sleep, and felt constantly fatigued. The physiotherapist gave her a set of graduated exercises, which she struggled through but which brought neither relief nor improvement. The pharmacist even clucked his tongue one day when she bought some over-the-counter sleeping pills. She hadn't known that people really did cluck their tongues but as soon as she heard the slight sound she knew what it was.

The principal of Marie's school signed a form for a medical leave of absence for her, but he obviously didn't understand why she would need it. After a year, she applied for a Disability Pension, which the insurance company finally grudgingly approved. She thought that that would be the end of it, but they seemed to want a re-evaluation every six months and she found that process to be exhausting, embarrassing, and somehow demeaning—"They don't believe me. They think I'm scamming the system—x-rays and CAT scans don't show anything, anyway."

Somehow, from an active, happy person, Marie had become a sorry woman whose whole life now revolved around her pain. How did that happen?

IDENTIFYING THE "OUTSIDE" MEMBERS OF THE DANCE COMPANY

Let's look at our case scenario and begin to identify the various participants in this intrusive, constant interaction with pain.

There are many obvious "outside" dancers, some of whom have fairly important roles: Marie's family doctor, and the three specialists; the physiotherapist; the pharmacist (and, for that matter, the checking clerk in the drug store)—these are the members of the medical and paramedical part of the dance troupe. Then there are the home care nurses and/or homemakers who do the brunt of the housekeeping.

Marie's family—her parents, brothers, and sisters (we don't know anything about them, but they are sure to be involved in some way); other family members; her friends; and perhaps her neighbors.

Next, we must remember all the people connected with Marie's profession—the principal of the school, her fellow teachers, and her pupils, who wonder what happened to their teacher and why she isn't with them any more.

The Disability Pension people are going to have a major, if periodic, impact, especially if they are going to continue to reevaluate her situation every six months.

And there are two people who are the crux of the whole outside troupe—Tim, and the drunk driver who caused the ghastly accident.

RELATING THE "OUTSIDE" MEMBERS TO THE EGO STATES WITHIN

Now let's take a look at the ego states within Marie. First we have "the patient"—the principal dancer who is deeply and irrevocably connected with the medical and paramedical counterparts on the outside.

Marie isn't used to being "a patient." She had led a vigorous, satisfying life with lots of activity and interests, and she was seldom ill. Furthermore, it was this vigorous life that she shared so importantly with Tim. Her self-image had never been that of an invalid, or indeed of a woman who was restricted in any way in what she wanted to do. To be so impaired now is intolerable to Marie, and yet she can't seem to do anything to change it. In such a situation her self-esteem will plummet, as indeed it already has.

This loss of self-esteem is exacerbated with every interaction— having the doctor say that the medication "should" be helping her; having the pharmacist cluck his tongue when she went for some sleeping pills. And the pitying looks from the girl at the check-out counter, looks that were mixed (Marie felt) with disdain, nearly caused her to lose whatever self-control she had, and burst into tears right there in the store.

Having been one who was always there to help others, she's now the one who has to ask for favors—a horrid, invidious change.

And when the Disability Pension people write to say that it is time for another "re-evaluation"—she just feels she *cannot* face them again. WHY, she asks herself, do they need to keep doing this? The only answer she can come up with is that they obviously don't believe her; they are, silently, accusing her of malingering or at least of making everything much worse than it actually is. Naturally, the Disability evaluators will say that they are only interested in anything that may have changed.

She tries not to think of what her life would have been like if the accident had never happened, but that, also, is too painful to contemplate; and yet her mind keeps going back to it, like one's tongue insistently finding a sore tooth.

Also, within herself, is the ego state of "wife"—the part of herself that was only married for seven years before this happened— and that part feels completely cheated. Will she ever be a "real" wife again?

And what about ever becoming a "mother"? At this point she cannot even imagine herself taking care of a child. The emotional pain which all of this creates will add to the physical pain a thousand-fold.

Marie was also a competent, highly-regarded "teacher"; no more does she fill that role. It seems to her that her principal can barely hide his disappointment that she has not "gotten over this little mishap." But the part of her that loved teaching, that knew how good she was at it, is still there within her, and is mourning the loss of her professional identity and her vocation. Her professional identity used to be the part of her that sustained her self-concept in so many ways. Now it has been eroded so badly that, instead of being a strength within her, it is one of the heaviest burdens.

These feelings of loss all add to her pain.

She even has a "guilty part" of herself—the part that reminds her constantly that it was *Tim* who was so badly hurt, not she. She didn't even realize that she was hurt until weeks later. This awareness creates even more self-doubt, adding another pound to the weight of her despair.

And despair has set in, for sure. She is at risk for a significant clinical depression, with all that that entails, including sleep problems, inability to focus and concentrate, forgetfulness, and—very important—the biochemical changes that take place within the body when severe depression gets a solid foothold.

Suicide? Something that, before the accident, she would never have dreamt of in a million years; but now—somehow not such a very unlikely idea.

Then there is her sense of herself within her family—"the daughter," "the sister," "the niece" or "the cousin." These used to be such vibrant ego states; now, they are shrinking and tarnished with her invalidism.

If she searches way down into her subconscious, she would also find the part of herself that was—is—furious that she was such a "stupid klutz" on the trampoline. (See? This *must* be all my fault, after all.)

There are two more ego states that are among the most important. The first we can call "the pain self"—that part of Marie which is completely involved with the experience of pain and its intrusion into her life, and there is also a very positive, healthy part—the Angry Self: not anger-turned-inward, which is depression, but rather an energy-giving "I-will-do-something-to-change-this" anger that can have the power to initiate and sustain change even in the most desperate of circumstances.

Well, *that's* quite a troupe:

"Outside" Dancers

family doctor
specialists
physiotherapist
pharmacist
drug store staff
principal of school
other teachers
pupils
homemakers and home care nurses
parents
family members
friends
Disability evaluators
neighbors
the drunk driver
Tim

"Inside" Dancers

the patient
the one who has to ask for favors
her only-married-seven-years self
the future mother
previously competent teacher
the depressed one
daughter
sister
cousin
former bright, happy friend
the 'positive-angry' self
the 'pain' self
the 'guilty-because-Tim-was-badly-hurt' self
her past 'klutz' self

There's little wonder that the chronic pain patient—as we can see in the case of Marie—becomes so enmeshed in the situation that his or her whole life gradually and inexorably comes to re-volve more and more around the pain.

We have identified many, if not all, of the Dancers in our sce-nario. Others may turn up as the Dance proceeds. Now—

WHAT ABOUT THE DIRECTORS AND CHOREOGRAPHERS?

Each of the Dancers—Inside and Outside—has a greater or lesser role in the life of chronic pain which Marie now leads. But which are those who really direct the whole scenario? Who are the di-rectors, who the choreographers?

In my experience, the directors' roles are usually taken by one or more outside participants, and the role of the choreographer comes from within the self.

For example, Marie spends a good deal of her time following the advice of her doctors, and less time (but which feels in many ways more devastating) dealing with the disability evaluators. It is literally true that these people now direct her life in very sig-nificant ways. She can't get along without them; and this—for someone who had been such an independent woman—is a mis-erable situation which is made even more miserable by Marie's conviction that these "directors" don't really believe that she *has* excruciating pain. So far, no one has been able to explain to Marie why her back, after being comfortable and highly functional for decades, should suddenly turn traitor.

Now that we have identified a possible director, which of Marie's states is the choreographer? To determine the choreogra-pher, Marie must ascertain which part of her organizes her in-ward responses to the daily situations of life, because this may be where change can begin. It might be that of "the patient," or "the depressed one." Every patient has his or her own way of inter-preting the choreographer's role.

S amantha quickly grasped the concept behind the metaphor and was pleased that there was some new approach to ex-plore.

She easily identified the directors—her neurologist and, in a more day-to-day role, her G.P. There were also the nitty-gritty hurdles that Dave seemed to direct for her, such as getting her to the doctor's, to the drug store, or to the Emergency Room.

When it came to the choreographer, however, she had her own very definite ideas about how to interpret that.

"It's *the pain itself*," she stated positively. "The PAIN is the choreographer. It dictates and decides my every movement—literally."

Who could argue with that?

THE PROGRESSION OF THE DANCE

In acute pain situations, the dance is carried on, by and large, with the self. Others may be drawn in for a specific part of the Dance (for example, the surgeon who performs the appendectomy), but their roles are limited to specific functions. Once the acute stage is over, the dance of acute pain intrudes very little into the day-to-day life of the person.

When pain becomes persistent, there are always more members of the company because the patient will continue to be involved with medical people in one way or another. There will be a family doctor or G.P. and one or more specialists, and perhaps a legally appointed consultant for some special purpose; there will be the pharmacist at the local drug store, probably a physiotherapist, and maybe a psychologist or a referral to a pain clinic.

The patient has long ago begun to spiral down that helpless/hopeless precipice. But if some creative way is found to interrupt this spiraling down, there is chance for significant improvement in the person's quality of life—as in the case of Charlie.

Charlie was injured at work; a lapse of attention, and a heavy piece of equipment came down on his foot. Luckily there were several other people around and he was extricated fairly quickly, but there was terrible deep, deep bruising of his calf and foot from the crushing; two of his metatarsal bones were fractured, and he had torn some ligaments in his ankle.

Charlie got good medical care and his leg and foot apparently got better, but the pain—instead of diminishing—

seemed to become more intense. At first he was quite philosophical about this, but as the days and weeks wore on, he began to get worried.

He went back to work, but his intake of analgesics went up and up. One of his coworkers recognized this and approached him directly. "Charlie, you should not be operating heavy machinery with all those pain killers in your body. You *know* that that's not a safe thing to do."

Charlie did know, but because the "pain killers" didn't kill the pain at all, he had convinced himself that it was okay. He said as much to his fellow worker.

"I don't think that's right," said his friend, doggedly. "I'm worried about you—and about those of us who work with you. What if you have another accident and one of US gets hurt?"

That stopped Charlie in his tracks. He couldn't even imagine how he would feel if he caused one of his fellow workers to be injured. "Maybe you're right," he acknowledged slowly, "But I don't know what to do about it—without the pills I couldn't function at all. And I've *got* to work."

Charlie was well into a persistent pain situation, and more and more people were being drawn into the Dance.

Luckily, he was referred to a pain clinic where he was greeted, and treated, with dignity and understanding—and firmness. The staff at the clinic were all very aware of the patterns that we have been describing here, and although their vocabulary would have been different, they understood how a sufferer's life often began to revolve around the pain. In their various ways, they helped Charlie to identify the different factors which affected his pain and his response to it—including the people involved—and he began to slowly climb back up the slope. Because his life was no longer focused completely on the pain (in other words, the choreography had changed), he gradually came off his medication and was able to go back to work safely despite the residual discomfort. Charlie was a man for whom it was vitally important to be a contributing member of society—it was an integral part of his self-image—and getting back to work was worth a lot to him.

It would be wonderful if all persistent pain patients were as lucky as Charlie but, unfortunately, most are not.

One day Samantha confided the events which brought her into my office for the first time.

"It was my mother and Dave," she told me. "They were on my back the whole time. I guess they heard about hypnosis and thought that it might work—nothing else seemed to be helping very much at all. So, to shut them up, I allowed my mother to phone and make the appointment."

She hadn't expected anything positive to come from it, and in fact thought that hypnosis was just hokey mumbo-jumbo anyhow; so she was quite surprised to find that, not only was she able to go into hypnosis with my guidance, she was also able to do it herself.

But it didn't help the pain when a headache really got going. *Nothing* helped the pain when a headache really got going.

So far we've been focusing on those Dancers who seem to be (in some sense) saboteurs, undermining the sufferer in some way, even though their intentions are good. It's important to also identify the Helpers.

Helpers—both from outside and from within—are unique because they have virtually no agendas of their own to maintain; they are able to do some kind of service or fill some role for their friend, family member, or other ego states without it being an imposition on the helpers' lives or roles.

Once again we must look both inside and outside. This takes a bit of determination, because many Dancers have dual roles— partly helper, partly saboteur.

In our next chapter we will approach this from the other direction, that is, from the perspective of 'what are the *roles*' rather than '*who* is in the cast.' Dual roles are probably many times more common than either the undiluted saboteur or the total helper.

PERTINENT POINTS FROM CHAPTER FOUR

We can begin to identify who the "Dancers" are, and who the "Director" or "Choreographer" might be.

The **director(s)** are very often from the medical or legal community.

The roles can come from inside (**ego states**) or outside.

The dance of pain is a **progression**—acute pain may lead into persistent pain which may then lead to chronic pain.

It is important to **interrupt the progression** at the **earliest possible** point.

WORKSHEET FOR CHAPTER FOUR

1. Identify the dancers—inside and out—in **your** scenario:

a. Outside dancers

b. Inside dancers

CHAPTER FIVE

NAMING YOUR PAIN PLAYERS

What Are the Roles?

THE MEDICAL "COMMUNITY"

As I stated in the last chapter, I think of the various members of the medical community as being among the Directors. After all, as doctors we truly DO 'direct' people to do this or to do that—always with the best of intentions, because we feel that we know what's best for the patient at that time, in that situation. (There are, of course, many solid arguments against this attitude, and I fully acknowledge them, but this isn't a book about doctors' bad attitudes, except insofar as how those attitudes affect and influence the choreography of pain.)

Let's start with the G.P. or Family Physician (not exactly the same thing, technically speaking, but close enough for our purposes). The "family doc" is usually the one who will know the family best and who will be in more constant communication with them. Generally speaking, consultants will speak directly to the patient and then communicate with the family physician, to whom he or she sends reports and advice for continuing care.

The family doctor will usually be the one to suggest specialists, prescribe medications, arrange for physiotherapy, and/or refer the patient to pain clinics. In these regards, then, family doctors truly are "Directors" in pain management—in our metaphor, in maneuvering the choreography.

It is usually the family doctor upon whom the patient depends most directly and most despairingly. He or she is front and center on the firing line of the patient's desperate search for relief. The problem is, usually the family doctor runs out of options fairly quickly and finds him/herself also pretty desperate and, after a while, despairing. Of course, these feelings are not in the same league of intensity as those felt in the patient; but they are nevertheless there and, I believe, are in large part responsible for the apparent wall which patients perceive and believe is there when they want and need to communicate with their doctors.

This may account for some of the apparent duality of saboteur/helper which is really epitomized in the medical support system. I like to believe that all my medical colleagues truly want to help; I also know that at times our *own* fears and frustrations nullify our best intentions.

Directing the directors, so to speak, are the specialists to whom the family doctor refers—surgeons of many subspecialties, neurologists, rehabilitation doctors, psychiatrists ("Horrors!" would say some people who still perceive a stigma), experts in pain management, perhaps even anaesthesiologists if, for example, the family doctor is wondering about nerve blocks.

The helper/non-helper schism here usually has something to do with the insularity of the specialists; one can only see them on referral, they almost always have watch-dog receptionists, and one cannot just "drop in" on them. In other words, there is limited availability and, although the patient knows that getting along without the specialist would be impossible, at the same time one might wish for a slightly more congenial interaction.

In the Suburbs of the Medical Community

Also dancing leading, or possibly directorship, roles are those in the neighboring areas. We've already mentioned many of them: pharmacists, physiotherapists, nurses, psychologists and other counselors, to name just a few. Seldom are these people in major directorship roles, but they do hold a particular place in the spectrum. For instance, their attitude has a significant impact on the patient (remember Mary's reaction to the tongue-clucking of the pharmacist). Nurses who are involved in pain management are very well educated about the manifestations of pain, and the intense psychosomatic response, but others may not be. Imagine the spin-off if the nurse-receptionist in the doctor's office didn't really think it was very important to schedule the chronic pain patient in to see the doctor that day. From an intellectual point of view, she may have been right; but from a psychological perspective it may have been that crushing blow that sent the patient into depression—the straw that broke the camel's back, as it were, or, in this case, the erosion of a last fragile support.

One of my chronic pain patients, with horrible low back pain and coccyalgia (pain in the tail bone) resulting from a work-related accident, felt very bad vibes from the several physiotherapists she had seen who were associated with the Workers' Compensation Board. After several years, she moved to a very small town and found, quite unexpectedly, a wonder physiotherapist who has brought her continuing and incremental relief since the very first appointment. She can now sit in a chair without pillows or squirming for the first time in years. She feels the physiotherapist has a major role in her pain choreography. This physiotherapist is a true "helper" dancer.

We must mention, for the sake of completeness, emergency personnel such as ambulance drivers, paramedics, firefighters, police officers and others who attend the injured at the scene of an accident or other trauma. Although they play a major director role at the time, that role quickly dances itself off stage once the patient is transported to a hospital or treatment center.

But because their involvement *is* so crucial at the time, their words and behavior can have a severe and long-lasting impact on the patient—for better or for worse. It might be interesting for our scenario patient, Marie, to go back with the help of a well-trained therapist (I cannot stress the "well-trained" strongly enough) and revisit, emotionally, the scene of the accident and the subsequent hours in the emergency room, waiting for news of Tim. Who was supporting her there? Did anybody bring her a cup of tea? Or just sit with her? She was so remote from her own injuries at that time that she didn't even realize she had any—that is, she was truly dissociated from her injuries and pain. I believe that the impact of those experiences stays with people for a very long time and DOES affect their own responses, both emotionally and physiologically, long, long after their wounds are apparently, theoretically, "healed."

Remember, we are talking about all aspects of pain in the context of chronic pain having a huge *suffering* component: the patient *suffers* such intrusion into his or her life. It is not hard, nor is it unrealistic, to trace much of the suffering to emotional factors. Emotions intensify and exacerbate pain, especially chronic pain. There is nothing imaginary about this.

So we see that, very often, the roles of the medical and paramedical community have to do with directorship. Everybody knows how risky it is for a performer to be mad at the director; it is a hundred times riskier to *show* that he or she is mad at the director—such performers might very well find themselves not performing for a while.

How much riskier again (a thousand times?) for a patient to be mad at the doctors, *when that patient still needs so much from those doctors*! Scary stuff.

Samantha had been to see her neurologist, in whom she had great faith. While many others in the medical community had upset her in the past, her family doctor and her neurologist were two people upon whom she knew she could rely, and be heard.

She had told him about coming to see me, and the work we were doing together.

"He raised his eyebrows," she said, laughing, "and told me to let him know how it was working out.

Obviously he doesn't expect much! But he *did* understand when I said that our work here was giving me some tools to use myself, and a bit of a different perspective, and that that felt good. He said that that was very important."

"Any changes in your medication?" I asked.

"No, I'm just to stay on the ones I'm on. I'm taking a lot, but he seems to think it's okay. I know he keeps looking for a good prophylactic."

Samantha's neurologist was one of those intuitive 'directors' that we all long for—one who truly listens to the chronic pain patient.

THE LEGAL MEMBERS OF THE DANCE COMPANY

The other group of involved people who frequently fill the directorship role is the legal/insurance/compensation/disability group.

And again, it is very hard to show any kind of anger to those
people that adjudicate you in some legalistic way, and upon whom
you are dependent for compensation, disability or pension bene-
fits.

In the eyes of the chronic pain patient, this 'legal community'
is almost always adversarial to them. That may or may not be
true and of course there are exceptions, as in everything, but generally that is the perception based on the experiences of the patients involved.

Let's take an example.

Mr. J. was, of all things, knocked off his horse.

He was horseback riding with a tour group. He and
seven other senior citizens (Mr. J. was 67 years old at the
time) were on a two week "Explore the Back Country!"
experience. On the day of his mishap, they were out on a
trail ride through more rugged country than he was used
to. Although Mr. J. had ridden horses since he was a lad,
his experience was more or less limited to rural pathways
or gently rolling hills.

As far as he can remember, because he was knocked out
for a few minutes, Mr. J.'s horse was bumped by another
more rambunctious mount and Mr. J. was pushed into the
branch of a pine tree which lifted him off the horse and
onto the rocky ground.

The tour guide had never had such a thing happen before and was not very experienced in emergency situations.
He even forgot that he had a cellular phone until one of
the other people in the group asked him to use it to call
for help.

Besides a mild concussion, Mr. J. sustained a commin-
uted fracture (many pieces) of his left femur. He was he-
licoptered out to the nearest hospital, a small 17-bed unit
in the little town where they were staying as a base for
their Back Country experience.

The doctor there stabilized Mr. J. and, because Mr. J.

also had a history of angina and a somewhat labile blood pressure, he was then sent to the large tertiary care hospital in the city where he lived.

That was three years ago. Mr. J. has never regained full use of his left leg, walks with the aid of a four-footed cane, and is well into a chronic pain syndrome.

Mr. J. is suing the tour company, the tour guide, and the doctor who first attended to him who, Mr. J. said, should have done something more at the time. Mr. J. also found that the medical insurance which he thought he had was invalid because he was out of the territory in which he was covered.

Mr. J. retained an aggressive young lawyer to handle his case. The tour company responded in kind and pulled up a big gun of their own. The doctor was covered by malpractice insurance and exonerated of any blame. The tour guide had a nervous breakdown and launched a counter-suit, which he originally lost and which is now under appeal.

Do you think all this action is doing Mr. J. much good, pain-wise?

He is angry at his lawyer, whom Mr. J. now thinks is not experienced enough; in addition to that, of course, he is angry at himself for choosing that lawyer; he cannot understand why the tour company doesn't just accept responsibility for the problem and pay up, and he is furious that the doctor got off "scot-free," although there was no evidence of any mishandling of the case within the confines of the small hospital in which the doctor worked.

Mr. J. sought a second legal opinion and was advised that the lawyer he had was doing his best, and to change over at that date would further prolong the whole process.

Now, we may wonder at the pros and cons of this particular case, but the fact remains that Mr. J. feels at the mercy of the legal system, that the medical/insurance systems have failed him, and that he is going to have a heart attack any minute. His leg gives him excruciating pain, particularly at night, and his lifestyle has been severely disrupted. Clearly, Mr. J.'s life—and his pain—are being directed by the legal and insurance systems.

It's not hard to see the overlapping of helper/saboteur in this convoluted situation. It's also not hard to appreciate how much the disruption adds to Mr. J.'s pain.

HOW ABOUT THE FAMILY?

If ever there was opportunity for intermingled helping and sabotage, the roles of the family exhibit these possibilities.

O ne day, Samantha and I were talking about her mother.

"Remember when you asked me if she was one of the dancers?" I asked.

"Yes, of course."

"How did you relate that to your mother's love for you?" I knew that Samantha was in no doubt about that, but that she often railed against what she perceived as overprotection.

"Well," she answered slowly, "I *don't* think it means that she doesn't care for me. I know how much she does. Maybe she cares too much?"

"And how might that express itself?"

"Probably it would look like—does look like—she was interfering. I often get really mad at her for that. But I know she needs to *do* something to feel that she's useful. So it comes across as a real intrusion but she's just wanting to help and she doesn't know any other way."

Of course, Samantha's interpretation was quite right. Mother was both a saboteur and a helper. Untangling these roles can be very difficult, but it's important to do so, so we spent the rest of the session discussing ways and means.

I often refer to family members and close friends, who want so desperately to help but are really undermining the person's own struggle for independence, as the "Beloved Saboteurs." The phrase always brings a smile of recognition and a nod of the head when I ask, "Who are the Beloved Saboteurs in your choreography?" Beloved Saboteurs have to be confronted with great tact and respect in order for the situation to change. This can be *very* difficult to do.

Although at times some family members may assume (or fall into) directorship roles, I think they are more often members of the troupe—and very important members, too.

Immediate family members are the most frequently involved, naturally. It's almost impossible for them NOT to be involved. The question always becomes, "What kind of roles are they dancing? Helpers? Beloved Saboteurs? Sometimes (sad to say), not-so-beloved saboteurs? Or—even sadder—nasty-minded saboteurs?" Luckily the latter category is rare. When it does exist, it is completely devastating.

Jackie and Lois are sisters. They both work in the same retail company—Jackie as receptionist to the vice-president and Lois as floor manager in one of the main departments.

Two years ago, Lois fell on the ice and cracked her pelvis. It was not considered a terribly dangerous injury, but it involved her being off her feet for a period of time to give the bone time to heal solidly. To all appearances, it *did* heal solidly and she went back to work.

After being back a few weeks, she began to experience shooting pains in her lower back and sometimes it felt as if her hips were not very firmly in their sockets. She was thoroughly investigated with all the latest in modern technology, and nothing abnormal was found to account for her discomfort. Her doctor advised that she go for some more physiotherapy, which she did. She said, bitterly, that all THAT accomplished was to make it hurt more.

Going to work became a major problem, because she was almost incapacitated by pain by about 11:00 a.m. As a result she was short-tempered with her staff and they began to complain about her. One day she was short-tempered with a customer, and that created a more immediate problem because the customer also complained—to the vice-president.

Now, there had always been antagonism between Jackie and Lois, from the time they were children. Jackie was the elder by two years, and everyone said that her nose was put out of joint when Lois was born. As for Lois, all through school she had had to endure being compared to Jackie, who was considered to be a very intelligent girl, was also very active in sports, and in her senior year in high school was president of the Student Council. Lois was considered to be neither particularly intelligent—although certainly passable—nor sports-minded, and she never aspired to any kind of elected office.

After high school, the two embarked on somewhat divergent paths, Jackie going to college and Lois getting right into the work force, where she proved to be a capable and reliable worker. In fact, she had risen in the ranks to be head of her department—the same firm which Jackie joined several years later.

To put it bluntly, the two women didn't like each other. Each thought the other was callous and self-serving. They put on a reasonable front of family solidarity in public, but in private they stayed as far away from each other as possible. When everyone at work began to commiserate with Lois, Jackie became quite jealous of the attention Lois was receiving, and when the complaints began to come in, she felt Lois was finally getting what she deserved.

With the final complaint by the irate customer, Jackie saw her opportunity. She spoke privately to her boss and, because she was in a position of trust with him, he listened carefully as she described Lois' character in less than complimentary terms. The end result was that Lois was put on mandatory leave of absence and instructed to get a psychological assessment.

For Lois, losing the position that had meant so much to her—she had no illusions about the likelihood of being accepted back on staff—increased her suffering a hundredfold and this was, of course, translated into an excruciating exacerbation of pain. Unable to endure it any longer, she made a serious suicide attempt. Although she recovered physically, she remained very depressed and under psychiatric care. Jackie, meanwhile, continued to rise in her company.

It's not very hard to recognize the roles of both Lois and Jackie in this *pas de deux*, which almost became a dance of death.

The foregoing is a combination of a couple of cases, partly to disguise them and partly because they do, in fact, exhibit very similar situations and both ended with suicide attempts.

In contrast, here is a case (not combined, this time) in which the roles of a very good friend and a husband were completely supportive.

Mrs. H. was in her early sixties when she joined my family practice. She had a very good friend who had been a patient of mine for several years and who suggested that Mrs. H. come to see me. Both women (and Mr. H.) were European and all had been in Europe during the Second World War.

Mrs. H. had been experiencing sudden attacks of excruciating, lancinating pain in her back and legs for years, but it was becoming much worse. She never had any warning and the pain would make her shriek. She had been investigated by several physicians, orthopedic surgeons, and neurologists and had been told, each time, that nothing was wrong.

She *knew* something was wrong. Her husband of many years knew it, too—he had seen her in pain over too long a time and he understood her character and personality very well. Although he had heard her described as 'hysterical' and 'psychoneurotic,' those terms did not describe his wife of three decades and he gave her every bit of love and support of which he was capable (and that was LOTS!).

I also knew her friend very well, from being her family doctor for many years, and I understood something about that lady: I knew that she would never have tolerated an hysterical friend. She would have told her to smarten up years before and if the friendship was disrupted because of that, well, so be it. Because none of that had happened, I listened very carefully as Mrs. H. described her situation.

During the war, Mrs. H. had been struck by shrapnel many times. She still had some of it in her body, and that was obviously one possible source of the pain. One also had to consider psychological factors. She described the pain as being like a bolt of lightning—"blitzkrieg," in fact. This was something that had to be explored. Was her pain some sort of posttraumatic stress disorder? Was she reliving World War II air raids?

We discussed this. Mr. and Mrs. H. were both willing

to delve into all such possibilities but I could see that neither gave the idea very much credence.

And I kept remembering that my common sense, down-to-earth patient of many years did not suffer fools—or hysterics—gladly.

On examination, I could not find anything out of the ordinary with Mrs. H. In particular, her neurological exam was within normal limits and her musculoskeletal system seemed strong.

I referred her to a specialist in Internal Medicine, outlining the case as I have described it above. He couldn't find anything wrong with her, either. We talked it over and I told him, "This may be a silly basis for wanting further investigation, but—"; and he listened carefully, and nodded, and we decided together to refer her to yet another neurologist.

The end result was that Mrs. H. had a benign tumor of the spinal cord. The nerves had been so stretched over the enlarging mass that any sudden shift or turn had caused the lancinating pain. The tumor was removed and her pain was removed with it.

So this was not really a case history of chronic pain syndrome, as it had seemed to be at the outset, because there was an identifiable cause for the pain which was eventually found. The point is that, without the supporting roles of her husband and friend in Mrs. H.'s pain choreography, she might have continued to suffer needlessly for much, much longer or even—worst case scenario—might not have received the appropriate treatment until it was much too late. True "Helper" dancers, indeed.

Think back to our hypothetical case of Marie and Tim, and recognize the roles of Tim and (although we don't know anything about them) the possible roles also of parents, siblings, and other family members. And think of Samantha and her mother. And think of the situation of someone you might know—even yourself—who is in chronic pain, and sort out some of the "dancers" and what their roles are. Helpers or saboteurs? Recognize that helpers may at times seem awfully pushy or even interfering, and saboteurs are often very caring and dedicated.

How About "The Others"?

Many other people may dance peripheral roles in the choreography: friends, business acquaintances, fellow workers. It's worth thinking about—occasionally putting the situation into this metaphorical context will clarify some aspects of it. Why is so-and-so behaving that way? How come what's-her-name doesn't visit me any more?

THE "EGO STATES" AS PRINCIPAL DANCERS

As one might expect, ego states are often principal dancers.

Samantha states positively that one of her inside dancers—the pain itself—is the choreographer. It is that part of her which is completely subjugated by the pain, which "dictates and decides my every movement—literally."

Many people speak in similar terms about an ego state (or states) which controls them when the pain hits. "It's as if that part of me '*takes over*' and I can't do anything about it. I just sort of sit back and watch it, as if I'm an observer. Sometimes it's almost as if I can *see* THE PAIN, watch how it behaves—makes me behave—and I have no control over that part of myself at all. Sometimes it's even kind of scary."

As I've mentioned, ego states are those diverse parts of ourselves that come to the fore in various situations. I said that we are slightly different people when we're in the office than when we're at home, different as parents than as friends, different as spouses than as colleagues. We bring to each of these situations the experience, knowledge, learning, intuition and behaviors which are appropriate. Those of us who are trained in medicine, for instance, or psychology or counselling or nursing or law are strongly advised NOT to enter into "dual roles" with our patients or clients. It muddies the waters. We want to keep our ego states separate in their own appropriate fields.

Sometimes, of course, it's unavoidable. In a very small town, the only doctor might be your neighbor and friend, and when you're sick, you turn to him or her also. But we do expect both parties to recognize the variation in these interactions, and to act appropriately. In other words, we recognize the different ego states: neighbor becomes doctor, friend becomes patient. There can be warmth and humor and caring, but there is also an acknowledgement of the other agenda and attention paid to it.

Which of the various ego states are likely to be leading dancers in the choreography of pain?

We listed many of them in our hypothetical case of Marie: let's go back to that, from this slightly different perspective.

The "patient" is probably the ego state which has the most interaction with the medical and paramedical community—inside and outside dancers in a repetitive *pas de deux* every time some medical need arises: renewing a prescription, getting sent to a specialist. Because it is a familiar dance, both parties know their roles well. Also because it is a familiar dance, both parties get very frustrated with it and sometimes one or the other tries to change the rhythm, which may cause great consternation on the part of the other partner. The paradox is that often both parties long to change the dance, but don't know how.

When pain persists and travels inexorably into the chronic state, there is always, at some level, anger. You'll remember that, in my definition of pain, I call it the body's way of expressing anger. Thus there is bound to be at least one ego state which is identified in some way with anger—with the controlling of it, with the suppression of it, with the exploding of it, with dealing with the aftermath of it.

The roots of anger are frustration, fear, intrusion and injustice, in ascending order from 'being mad' to raging fury. A chronic pain patient may therefore have several ego states which are in some way identified with anger. If we are to ameliorate that patient's pain, dealing with the anger is a crucial part of the process. We'll talk more about this in the next couple of chapters.

Loss of a job or job status will evoke another ego state. From being a competent, active contributor to the work force, the pain patient may have become totally dependent on a disability pension or worker's compensation. Thus these ego states are the ones which dance with the legal/insurance/pension people and those can be very difficult and tricky dance sequences.

Let's say we have a woman who was assaulted in some way on the job. Her injuries involved a possible broken jaw, missing teeth and squashed nose, and her glasses were shattered; one wrist was badly sprained in trying to ward off the attacker and she had bumps and bruises all over.

She recovered from all these but was left with continuing facial pain, which she described as "unmanageable" and which prevented her from doing her job as a receptionist.

Of course she would be highly involved with the legal and compensation people right from the beginning and all was probably rosy in the early days; but when her pain persisted, the compensation board began to balk and eventually told her that she had received all she was going to receive. Can't you just imagine the intricasies of this dance, both sides jockeying for position and doing a shuffling two-step back and forth as they presented their arguments?

There is also the *loss* of the ego state that used to be competent—or at least, the pushing down of that part of oneself because it is no longer functional. People often don't recognize that this leads to a grief reaction—perfectly reasonable under the circumstances but so often misunderstood as whining or self-pitying. In some situations, there is also grief for 'what might have been' but now perhaps never can be, such as motherhood or some sort of championship or just the positive pleasure of having a fulfilling job throughout many years of one's life.

One of the most devastating of ego states is one that is associated with Guilt. This partner can dance with a whole slew of other participants, both inside and outside. There may be an intermezzo or two with the boss, for instance, or a fellow worker or some other person/people whom the sufferer believes has been let down. Guilt relating to a spouse or other family member (remember Marie and Tim) is extremely common; very often there are quarrelsome, discordant dances related to guilt and to the anger underneath it (anger on both sides).

From the perspective of the outside partner, these emotions are bewildering; it is dreadful to be angry at someone whom you love, who is suffering pain, and this bewilderment is a dilemma which can lead straight to a massive Guilt ego state in the outsider, too.

Inside Guilt may dance around depression, humiliation, grief, fury, loss of self-esteem, fatigue, insomnia, anxiety, and almost any other emotion you might think of. It is an invidious, dangerous inside saboteur, but it's not hard to see where it may have come from.

And then of course there are the ego states which evolve from the new situation—the long-suffering state, the risk of the martyr state, the ego state which stays home rather than goes out into the workaday world. These are the parts of the self that may become involved in "secondary gain" situations. There has to be *some* relief; sometimes it can be found in new consideration from a spouse, more attention from friends, or the opportunity to break with old dull routine and learn some new skill or pasttime, odd as it may seem to couch it in those terms. Remember that secondary gain is NOT related in any way to malingering or deceiving; it is the psyche's way of finding something positive, somewhere, in that otherwise awful situation.

Add all these to the roles of the outside participants, and you suddenly have an awful lot of dancers on the stage.

Samantha had come in with her usual wonderful smile. I had been away and hadn't seen her for three weeks. "How're things?" I asked.

"Oh, fine—but Dave has left me."

"Left you?" I was flabbergasted. She always spoke of their relationship as being the strongest, most supportive framework she had. And why wasn't she in tears? "Can you tell me about it? What happened?"

"I don't really know. He tells me that he still loves me very much, but he needs some space. He's staying with his mother."

She had herself in tight check—still no tears, still the wide smile in place. It was her way of coping.

Time went on, the hours and the days passed.

Samantha kept me up to date as we continued with our sessions. They spoke on the phone frequently, went out to dinner, and in a few weeks he was back. Finally, tentatively, they began to approach their feelings more directly. And a different kind of communication—a new dance—began.

"He told me that it seemed as if I didn't need him any more," Samantha said. "I seemed to be doing so much more on my own—seemed so much more independent—" her voice trailed off.

"So you two are creating a whole new relationship," I observed. "This will be very interesting."

"Yes," she said, somewhat pensively, "I know. Because now that I've begun to understand things differently, I know I must continue to go forward. And I will."

An old secondary gain situation—gain for both—had been upended. This new scene was scary, but exciting and full of promise.

PERTINENT POINTS FROM CHAPTER FIVE

Directors are usually in the medical and legal communities.

There are some special roles ("short solos!") danced by, for example, emergency room personnel and/or paramedics.

Outside players are extremely important—the dance with them often intensifies the pain through **stress;** this applies particularly to **legal** roles.

The **main outside dancers** are usually **family** and significant others.

There are both **helpers** and **saboteurs** and often these are **dual roles.**

Ego states are **usually lead dancers** but can at times assume directorship roles.

The **choreographer** may be inside or outside, and may be THE PAIN itself.

"Secondary gain" is a normal phenomenon and is **not the same** as malingering.

WORKSHEET FOR CHAPTER FIVE

1. Once again, identify the ego states in your own situation and how they relate to the outside players, but this time, particularly with respect to helpers and saboteurs:

2. Do you recognize some dual roles?

3. How might you "accentuate the positive and eliminate the negative" in those dual roles?

CHAPTER SIX

YOUR PERSONAL PATH TO WELL-BEING

How to Change the Dance

ACCEPTING THE CONCEPT

The first step toward changing The Dance of chronic pain is to accept the concept.

Remember, we are not talking about magic relief from pain—or any other kind of magic, for that matter. We're talking about a metaphor that describes, often in dismally accurate terms, a whole set of interactions.

We're talking about acknowledging that chronic pain invariably draws into its web many people other than the patient, and many ego states within the patient. All of these other people, sometimes separately and sometimes not, interact with the various aspects of the pain patient's psyche; it is these interactions which we have termed "The Dance."

Change almost always happens slowly and begins in small ways, especially when one wants to change a situation that has gone on for years. I believe that it's best to look toward making very small changes first—little shifts in awareness, in interpretation, in response. (That's how it will happen anyhow—we may as well align ourselves with the subconscious!) Once such little shifts have begun to happen, everything else begins to change too—as in any system, when one thing changes, everything else has to shuffle around to accommodate to that. In time, one can look at the situation and say "Hey! things *are* different!"

The concept, then, is that all of these folks, outside and inside, have roles to dance in the situation and some of these roles are less than helpful, if not downright sabotaging. By the same token, some saboteurs are inevitable, and one has to work around them, too.

IDENTIFICATION

We can begin to apply what we discussed in the earlier chapters: Who *are* the directors and the dancers? Who have the leading roles? Who *is* the choreographer?

To get started on this, I usually suggest that the patient get a big piece of paper and start writing down whose role is which, as in the Worksheet from Chapter Four. One can either list the dancers—inside and out—and attach roles to them, or list the roles and identify the dancers that fill these roles: doctors, legal players, friends and family, and one's ego states.

For someone whose pain began with a work-related injury, often the workers' compensation personnel (and these can be MANY!) are part of the dance; so, too, will be the boss(es) and fellow workers.

For victims of other kinds of trauma, such as motor vehicle accidents, then the other driver(s), any passengers, lawyers and perhaps law enforcement officers will have important roles. For the victim of violent crime, the perpetrator, police and Victims' Assistance can be added to the company.

Jack, our next hypothetical patient, was attacked at work by a fellow employee who suddenly "went off the deep end" one morning.

> Jack was hit from behind and slammed into a wall, knocking himself out and sustaining a concussion. His neck snapped back, similarly to what would have happened if he had been rear-ended in a car accident. Fellow workers subdued the other man and called the police, who took several minutes to arrive on the scene. In the

meantime, Jack had regained consciousness and had been helped onto a chair, where he sat holding his head in his hands.

The ambulance had also responded to the police call and, when the paramedics arrived, they were horrified to find that Jack had been moved and left no doubt in anyone's mind that that may have been a dangerous thing to do. He was taken to the hospital where he spent the night and was released the next day. Later, he wrote a note of appreciation to the ER staff, particularly one nurse who had been assigned to him and had carried out her nursing duties expeditiously, no nonsense, but with obvious concern for her patient. His own doctor had come to the emergency room to see him and confer with a neurologist who also happened to be there on call.

Jack recovered from the concussion, but six months later, with the law suit still being wrangled over because of the mental status of the attacker, his doctor classified him as suffering from "post-whiplash syndrome," warning that the pain and dysfunction might last for a very long time, even years. (This tactic of predicting future suffering to patients is, in itself, potentially very sabotaging. Although it is done with the best of intentions, including informed consent, a person in pain is in an altered state of consciousness and may receive such communication in an almost post-hypnotic suggestion mode.)

Well, that's enough to give us a good start. If YOU were Jack, how would you identify the chorus and principals in his dance? To which roles would you assign them? What are the emotional ego states which are bound to be included here?

For everyone, there will inevitably be those omnipotent doctors and paramedical personnel, physiotherapists, nurses, counselors of various kinds, as well as family and friends and neighbors.

Then, all those parts of oneself which express the various emotions; one's role in the family, at work, at school (if a student), as a friend; the part of that patient who suffers the most from the pain, physically; and all the other parts of the psyche that are personal.

Write them out, all of them. Identify everybody, every aspect, you can think of. Swallow your pride and ask your nearest and dearest to contribute what they might be able to see, but to which you may be too close. Avoid arguing or defending yourself—there is no need for that. At least for now, accept what they might have to tell you.

Then assign each identified part a role on the dance team. Identify which parts interact most often with which other parts. Who takes charge of things, when, and under what circumstances?

It's very important to clarify these roles, because the next step will involve modifying them in some way, and it's very hard to change things until you know what it is that you want to change.

MODIFICATION

Next big question: *Where can one begin to intervene?* Where can one find the first opportunities for modification?

One logical place to begin looking is in the lists of dancers who have now been identified.

For starters, is there a member of the troupe whose function is now finished, but who is still just sort of hanging around backstage?

Let's go back to Jack. Maybe the fellow workers who helped him to a chair can be eliminated from the dance floor? Nope, too important—Jack still wonders whether he would be having all these problems if they hadn't moved him. Oh, he knows that their *intentions* were of the best, but nevertheless—.

How about the fellow workers who stood back, or scurried for safety? Uh-uh; maybe if they'd DONE something, then Jack wouldn't have been so badly hurt.

Wait. There was the nurse in the ER, who was so very professional but at the same time allowed him to see her concern—but we wouldn't want to push her out of the scene, she's one of the positives! Well, then, maybe give her a bigger role for a while, and let the other ER staff, nurses, lab techs, and x-ray staff ease out of the *corps de ballet.* Yes, that might work— a little shift in emphasis, strengthening a good feeling and releasing those who certainly have no more involvement right now. (You didn't think there *was* still involvement? The chances are higher that Jack was hanging on to every single aspect of that day, not necessarily consciously but more likely subconsciously.) Anyway, we've already said that we start with *little* shifts.

Another way to start the shifts, as I mentioned earlier, is by having one of the strong ego states inside gently confronting one of the outside dancers, who is in some way sabotaging. This is extremely difficult to do for some folks, and may be almost impossible unless it is undertaken in the most benign circumstances. Best NOT to confront the doctor angrily when other parts of yourself feel so very dependent upon that doctor. Start small. Practice.

Maybe, for instance, if your next door neighbor is driving you crazy because she is always "popping over" to see if there's anything she can do for you, you could *give* her something to do for you. "Betty, could I ask you to mail some letters for me? I'll have them ready by tomorrow after lunch." Then if this is accomplished, it might be easier to say, "Thanks so much. It's good to know that I have such wonderful neighbors. I'll call you the next time something comes up." You could go on to explain that right now, you're working on rearranging your daytime schedule because you want to figure out which are your most productive times of the day, so that you can make the most of them. This involves short cat naps to recharge your batteries, so you're asking everybody NOT to phone or drop in during the weekdays until you get this sorted out. You might add that on the weekends, when Bob's home, he can let people know if you're feeling up to visiting. (This also gives Bob a slightly different emphasis.)

When you begin to get the hang of it, then modifying some of the small, more inconsequential, situations becomes rather fun, and it's good practice for the time when bigger modifications have to be tackled. It gives a sense of being back in control.

"My boss phoned again yesterday. He keeps asking when I'm going to be able to come back to work. As if I wouldn't be back tomorrow if I could!" Samantha, usually so controlled and self-contained, had tears in her eyes—tears of frustration, I knew.

"How did you respond?"

"I told him I'd think about it. I know that that's just a cop-out, but I keep thinking that maybe I *can* go back, just part time. . . ." Her voice trailed off as she looked at me. "Yeah, I know," she continued miserably. "I'd be back in the same state as when I left, in about two weeks."

"So?" My eyebrows were well up on my forehead as I looked at her quizzically. I was beginning to understand more of how she ticked.

"Well, I'll think about it for a couple of days," (she wasn't looking at me) "and then I'll call him back."

When she returned the next week, she had her façade firmly in place: the bright, breezy Samantha. Oh-oh, that indicated trouble.

"Well, I was thinking it over, and I decided I can go back two afternoons a week. That way I can get in 10 or 12 hours a week, and it'll help a lot with the finances, and I'll sort of keep my hand in."

"Mm-hmmm," I said, as noncommittally as I could. Two afternoons didn't compute to 10 or 12 hours, and she knew it.

"I'll see how it goes," she continued doggedly.

"Okay."

Smile bright, chin high, she left the office.

By the next week, things were obviously not going as well as she had hoped. She'd had a couple of major bouts of pain and hadn't been able to get through the work. She told me that she had decided to ask a colleague/friend to take on some of the work. They could do it together.

But within a very short time, it all broke down. Her neurologist had told her in no uncertain terms that she was *not* to go back to work, when she had last seen him. "I guess he was right. I just couldn't do it. I'm wondering if I'll ever be able to do it again."

This was an opening, and luckily I recognized it. "You sound as if your self-image is taking a bit of a beating."

She nodded. The façade was gone. "If I can't work, *Who am I?*"

Suddenly we were catapulted into a whole new area. Her professional, working self was the ego state that she identified as epitomizing who she was, justifying her existence. This was, in fact, the antidote ego state to that one which blamed herself for having migraines.

We had a lot of work ahead of us.

LIFESTYLE CHANGES

Other areas which need modification have to do with lifestyle, and these are very important. If you read the research and literature reviews (Chapter Nine) you will recognize how often lifestyle change is mentioned as an essential factor in bringing about relief—relief, of course, in the *suffering* component in the agony of chronic pain.

Regulated times for sleep, eating and activities (I won't say 'exercise'—it's such a bad word!) are very important. When one has so much to cope with, appropriate structure of the day and night can make all the difference between coping reasonably well and coping poorly. When we're considering lifestyle changes, then we're talking about changing the dance patterns which reflect those areas. This usually involves different ego states: as examples, we might have the part of one which experiences the insomnia and rails against it, the part who gets fatigued so quickly with any form of activity, the part who either doesn't want to eat at all because "life isn't worth it anyway" or the one who eats all the time because "to hell with it, you've got to have *something* to live for."

How to start modifying these things? Start, again, with something easy. The only person who knows which is the easiest area to tackle is the pain sufferer him/herself: not the spouse, or the family, or the doctor, or the workers' compensation appeal board. Of course he or she might start off by saying, "It's no good, I can't change any of those things." However, with patience and empathy and endless encouragement *and* firmness, that person can almost always be caringly bullied into changing. Of course, it is always true that no one else can make changes for us. We have to do it ourselves. And it is also always true that, at least on some level, patients would like us to make their changes for them, and that we would, if we could. But we can't. And this is a good thing, because who can have a feeling of accomplishment if someone else does all the work? And when, during one's life, would a sense of accomplishment be more important than at a time when all control seemed to be taken away?

Sandra, a chronic back-pain sufferer, used to be a good sleeper, but since her bike accident two years ago, she has suffered increasingly with insomnia. Like most insomniacs, she clock-watches. Usually she finally falls asleep about five a.m., then feels terrible when the alarm goes off at seven o'clock.

Although she is still able to maintain her job as a salesperson at a local camera store, she's becoming more and more terrified that the insomnia will take this last vestige of pride away from her. Already she had been questioned by the boss on a couple of occasions because she looked so tired. "It's just the pain in my back," she told him. But she knew that the pain was always much worse when she hadn't been able to get any sleep (there are good physiological reasons for this).

Motivation is a great thing, and the threat of losing one's job unless something changes is a great motivator. Sandra recently went to the sleep lab at the university and was amazed to find that she did, in fact, sleep for short stretches frequently through the night. All in all, she got about six hours' sleep. That should be enough, she thought, to carry me through my day, so why am I so tired?

Well, she's tired partly because coping with chronic pain is exhausting, and partly because, with her clock-watching, she had convinced herself that she wasn't sleeping at all.

As a first step, she has agreed to turn the clock to the wall. The first night she did this, she spent the night wondering what time it was; and the second night; and the third. But a couple of nights ago she fell asleep within about half an hour of going to bed and, to her utter astonishment, she woke up when the alarm went off.

She knows that this augurs well for the possibility that she *can* get into a better sleep cycle. Right now her motivation is high, so let's hope she keeps on with it.

Sandra made a very small change: turning the clock to the wall. From such little shifts, major changes evolve.

Similarly, other lifestyle changes can be addressed. Activities are often best resumed with a detailed and personal timetable. One person may only be able to take an extra turn around the living-room. Go with that. Take the extra turn each day for a week, then take two turns. Manage that for a week and then take three.

Pretty soon that person can take three turns, twice a day. Next step is walking to the end of the driveway, which involves a short flight of stairs down from the front door—and up again!

There are people who find that their pain is relieved by exercise, once they get going, and this may be the case more often than we think. It makes sense—with the exercise there is a greater blood flow to the muscles; any buildup of lactate within the muscles will be taken away with the increased circulation.

Making lifestyle modifications involves a different kind of 'dance routine'—a different choreography—for that part of one's daily life. Therefore, it may involve ascertaining *who is the choreographer* for this scene. Inside or outside? There may even be a special choreographer for these situations, such as a counselor (outside) or an internal self-helper (inside).

The routine of going to various doctors is another potential area for change. Sometimes this can take the form of a contract, written or verbal, which may include opportunities for telephone discussion under certain conditions. Such a contract will often ease the burden for both doctor and patient IF it is made through mutual agreement. No patients want to have their doctors mad at them; no doctors want to be mad at their patients.

Contracting may be a way to avoid unnecessary conflict and hard feelings. A good example of how contracting works is the case of Harriet in Chapter Seven.

MEDICATION

I haven't spoken much about medication. Doctors usually feel that analgesics play such a limited role in chronic pain syndromes that they are best discontinued; all they do is upset the gastrointestinal system. They may have a more important role in some cases where flare-ups of a chronic state (e.g., arthritis) clobber a patient for days or weeks.

Some medications are to be avoided whenever possible (e.g., sleeping pills and major tranquillizers). Some have a more obvious role—muscle relaxants, antidepressants, and occasionally, anxiolytics. As many pain victims know, antidepressants can help restore normal sleep cycles, especially when taken in very small doses. This will also relieve some of the pain. The newer families of antidepressants—SSRIs (serum serotonin re-uptake inhibitors) and

SNRIs (serotonin and noradrenalin re-uptake inhibitors) seem particlarly good for this, as do some of the old tried-and-true groups, the tricyclics. I'd like to emphasize the small dosage. We're not talking here about taking the medication to relieve depression but rather to ease the distress of pain. If depression is also a factor, then that's a different story. Of course, this is from my own perspective.

Samantha and I were talking about this business of most analgesics being virtually useless. She was positively bristling (although, of course, very courteous).

"This will probably always be a very thorny issue for me," she said firmly. "*Many* people that I have talked to with chronic pain *firmly* believe that—even despite many years of 'not being prescribed the *right* pain killer'—there is one out there, somewhere; the doctors just can't find it.

"You've mentioned polypharmacy," she went on, "and I believe that many people self-medicate huge amounts because most doctors don't understand pain and are unwilling to explore this. And what about the back-pain patient who has been told to exercise but it *hurts* too much even to do a little bit? With the *right* pain pill perhaps that person can 'hold' the pain enough to start an activity routine—what about breaking the 'pain/can't do it/more guilt/tension/more pain' cycle?"

I had been pontificating, and she had caught me at it.

For those who have been on hefty doses of analgesics, including over-the-counter medication, for an extended period of time, I believe it's best to wean off slowly. Even though doctors believe that these medications may not be doing much good, as far as relieving the pain is concerned, nevertheless the body has become used to them and needs time to withdraw gracefully.

Above all, this must be done in collaboration with one's doctors. Going off medication that you have been on for a long time is *not* a do-it-yourself project. People find that the dance routine between themselves and their doctors changes radically when they decide to quit their pills. Be prepared for a whole new interaction. *And* be prepared for a whole new emotion: a sense of independence.

PAIN RELIEF TECHNIQUES*

Chronic pain sufferers know far more about pain relief techniques—which ones work and which ones don't—than those who have never suffered in that way.

Being on the outside can never equate with what it's like on the inside. So it seems pretty presumptuous of someone like me, who has never experienced chronic pain, to be suggesting various ways to deal with it.

In my own defense, I have more than twenty years of experience in helping chronic AND acute pain sufferers to relieve much of the distress (although, as I've said, not always the sensation itself) that accompanies pain.

My plea is that you—whoever is reading this book—read it in the context of the choreography, the inevitable interactions between people and situations when one's life revolves around pain. Dislocating the previous framework, dismantling previous conceptions and attitudes, will allow a new perspective to emerge. When we change the staging and the set, The Dance has to change, too.

1. Mechanical Measures

To reiterate, the well-known 'mechanical measures' for relieving pain include physiotherapy of all kinds; heat, cold, splints, and supports; graduated, personalized exercise and activity regimes. Sometimes it is important to restrict movement, at least for a time; other times it is important to continue moving no matter what.

What's different about this in our metaphor? Recognizing the roles of external and internal members of the company.

The external ones are usually easy: mostly they are connected to the medical and paramedical community: doctors, nurses, physiotherapists, occupational therapists, massage, perhaps even the people who supply prostheses. Their roles are well defined. No one is in much doubt about that.

The internal dancers are the ones that fascinate us here. Some important questions to ask here might be, "Which ego states are presently interacting with the external roles?" "*How are you go-*

---

*Note: many of these have also been described in my earlier books, although not in the context of choreography.

ing to change that?" "*Who* would be able to interact better—less painfully, less emotionally, less despondently; *who* may be more motivated and secure?"

Obviously this requires a perusal of the troupe. Perhaps the director needs to 'retire' some dancer and put another in his/her place. If this all sounds very dissociative, it is. But then, as we've said before, pain is a dissociative experience. The advantage lies in taking control of the dissociation.

So let's suppose that the ego state which has been interacting with the physiotherapist, for example, has been the "grit-your-teeth-and-get-on-with-it" ego state—the one who is determined to get through by sheer will power. Perhaps it's time to let that part step aside (he or she has been on stage for a long time) and instead ask the "nobody-is-going-to-tell-ME-what-to-do" self to get involved. This should make for interesting dialogue between the physiotherapist and the insider. But it just might work—if that insider can listen and adapt the physiotherapist's suggestions in a way that makes sense.

Similar reappraisals may be of benefit in other areas (e.g., activities, or "who" wears the splint). Remember that angst often creates more pain. If someone (or a part of someone) is champing at the bit because he or she has to wear 'some contraption,' that agitation is very likely to be expressed by even more pain. Explore!

Here is another case.

Dorothy had sustained a terrible fracture of her left leg, including her knee, while skiing. Of course, she was enraged at herself for the accident to begin with, which she attributed to sloppiness on her part. "I should have known better," she kept muttering. "I *did* know better! Why, oh why did I go down that stupid slope when I was so tired?" On and on she ranted at herself. In the hospital, they said that she even did it in her sleep.

Dorothy was the sort of person to whom being in shape was of utmost importance, and that was part and parcel of looking her best at all times. Consequently, when she was told that she would have to wear a brace on her leg for at least four months, she nearly had a fit. "I can't wear that awful-looking thing!" she gasped. "*I can't!*" But she had to. The only alternative would have been to have her leg completely immobilized in a cast, or to have it in traction, slung up above her head, for weeks and weeks and weeks. That would have been even worse because she would not have been able to get around at all and she had to get to her job.

Her inward-directed rage magnified her pain. She blamed it on the splint itself, the orthopedic surgeon who put her leg back together again—projecting her anger anywhere and onto anyone except where she could not bear to direct it—at herself.

When the choreography metaphor was first explained, she laughed harshly and said "Oh, sure! *That* would help, alright! I don't think so!" However, with considerable persuasion, she began to consider it less antagonistically.

Eventually she determined that it was the "proud-of-my-body" part of her that had to wear the splint and hated it so much. This made sense, of course. After considerable deliberation, she agreed to find out what would happen if the "I'm-going-to-make-sure-my-leg-heals-as-perfectly-as-possible" part of her took over that chore. Then she could get back to being "proud-of-my-body."

She could hardly believe the change in herself. Suddenly, wearing the splint was useful and therefore completely acceptable. Much of the extra pain which wearing it had caused, ebbed away. Eventually she dated her sudden rapid healing from that point.

As you can see, applying this metaphor can take a fair amount of imagination on the part of both patient and therapist. However, when it comes to chronic pain, *every* avenue is worth exploring.

2. Relaxation and Similar Techniques

Again, to reiterate: relaxation techniques, yoga, meditation and similar pursuits often bring an unexpected level of comfort. The single greatest factor is the *release of muscle tension*. Because all pain, whatever its origin, has some muscle tension component, simply easing that tension will ease that component of the pain. It undoubtably played a part in Dorothy's scenario, above.

The most effective and also the easiest of all the relaxation techniques, in my mind, is the Breathing technique. An added advantage is that you can do it anywhere because everybody breathes, and we all sigh from time to time.

You simply find the most comfortable (or least uncomfortable) place in the body. Then, using the creative imagination that we all have, visualize or feel yourself drawing in comfortable feelings from the comfortable part, as you breathe in. It's a little bit like sucking something up with a straw. Then, as you breathe out, you imagine yourself sending all that comfortable feeling right through your body; and while you're breathing *in* comfort and relaxation, you are also breathing *away* the pain and tension—pushing it out and replacing it with those comfortable feelings.

With a little practice, you can become very good at this. Then you'll have a new skill to ease pain, all ready, any time you might need it.

Some people who have one particular part of the body that always seems to be in spasm, or some kind of tension, have discovered that they can focus on that part of the body and deliberately make it *tighter*. This may seem ridiculous, but it often works. They tighten that particular muscle group, tighter and tighter, and more and more tense, until they can't GET it any tighter, then—as if they were releasing a huge balloon that was about to burst—they let go of ALL the tension at once. It is as if, in this way, they are able to release all the underlying residual tension at the same time as they release the tightness they have just added. Very interesting.

Also, some kinds of stretching exercises help to relax muscles. Athletes stretch all the time, of course, when they "warm up" before a game or a race. Stretching is also part of some of the yoga positions that can bring relief when they are done properly.

Let's get a dialogue going here between two key inside players, OUCH and EASE: OUCH is the ego state that feels the part of the pain due to tension (probably because OUCH is very tense him/herself). We'll make it *her*self here, just for simplicity. EASE is the ego state that feels some relief if the pain sufferer engages in relaxation or stretching activities.

OUCH: Hey! What do you think you're doing? That hurts!

EASE: Oh, for goodness' sake, I'm just doing a little bit of stretching. It's good for me.

OUCH: Well, stop it. I've got enough pain without you adding to it with your silly yoga stuff.

EASE: Come on, now—you know you felt better after we went swimming the other day.

OUCH: That was different. That was in the water and (self-righteously) the physiotherapist told me that the cool water helps my circulation, which helps to make my back more comfortable. And besides (warming up to her subject), the physiotherapist said that when I exercise in water, it's a non-weight-bearing kind of exercise and that's *good* for me.

EASE: Sure! All that's true. But it's also true that when I stretch gently, it helps to lengthen out all those muscle fibers that are all knotted up, so it feels better. Come on (wheedlingly)—just a little stretch?

OUCH: No. *OUCH!* Hey! Stop that!

EASE: (Demurely) Oh, sorry.

OUCH: (Grumbling) Yeah, I bet.

EASE: Does that feel better now?

OUCH: Of course it feels better n—oh-oh. I get it. You made me stretch after all, and now it feels better. Right?

EASE: Well, it *does* feel better, doesn't it?

OUCH: Yes, but it's an underhanded trick, just the same.

EASE: Mea culpa. Now, just a *teeny* little stretch, again?

OUCH: (Smiling inside despite herself) Some people are never satisfied.

Well, flights of fancy are kind of fun, but you get the general idea. There is so often one part of us that resists doing something, and another part that is willing to explore. Let the part that is willing to explore lead the way from time to time.

There is another important aspect to relaxation/meditation types of activities that is not always mentioned, and that is the emotional release of tension which so often accompanies these techniques. This is just as important as the physical release and, in many cases, probably even more so. When there is a lot of internal wrangling going on, as is always the case with chronic pain, there is bound to be a great deal of emotional tension. This will, in turn, prompt the release of hormones and neurotransmitters (biochemical substances which facilitate mind/body communication) which usually add to the pain in one way or another. It might, for example, interfere with sleep and thus exacerbate the release of Substance P*; or it might create more anxiety which, in turn, causes more tension.

The Relaxation Response has been studied now for decades. The general consensus is that, with such calming, there is an increased sense of well-being which in turn promotes comfort.

We also know that there are some people who feel they can *never* relax, and who even get angry at the suggestion that they do so. I think they get angry because they are so frustrated that they cannot seem to do this "thing" which everyone talks about so glibly.

Remember that we are talking about the release of muscle tension that comes with all of these techniques, and that the mind often remains very active while we are engaged in them. (This may be different for those who are skilled in the various forms of meditation in which the goal is to let conscious thought recede, but this can take years of practice and discipline and not all of us are as good at those.) If you get pleasure from listening to music, incorporate that into your relaxation times; if you like to watch funny movies, by all means follow that route. Norman Cousins, in his book *Anatomy of an Illness*, described watching old Marx Brothers movies and laughing his head off, and afterwards he experienced a relief of pain and also improvement of some of the laboratory tests (such as sedimentation rate) which were used to monitor his disease.

This would definitely be an example of the release of *emotional* tension.

3. Hypnotic Pain Relief Techniques

Using hypnosis and self-hypnosis to discover ways to become more comfortable is, as some of you may know, a favorite approach of mine.

Let me say a few words about hypnosis, first, because there is still so *much* misinformation and misunderstanding about this very simple, normal phenomenon. Myths and fears abound.

---

*Substance P is a hormone that is involved in the perception of pain, and is produced during periods of interrupted stage-4 sleep.

There's nothing magical about hypnosis. Hypnotic techniques are simply ways to focus attention, and when we do that, it's as if we take a step away from what we would otherwise be paying attention *to*. And we all do it all the time. Do you recognize any of these situations?

You're engrossed in a good book and all of a sudden you realize that you should have started to get dinner ready half an hour ago.

You're in an important board meeting and you suddenly realize, horrified, that the president is asking you to respond to something and you have no idea what anybody has been saying since Joe started mumbling on and on and on about his "little ideas to put some spark back into the project."

Your kids are so immersed in the TV that they haven't heard you call them, for the third time, to get their homework done.

You're driving down the highway and you suddenly realize that you've gone miles past your turn-off.

You turned off the alarm and turned on the radio and you've been listening to it—NOT asleep—and it's 8:06 and what has *happened* to the time since 7:30?

These are all spontaneous hypnotic experiences. But they're so commonplace and everyday that we don't think anything of them, and we certainly don't call them hypnosis, we call them "daydreaming" or some similar phrase.

Learning how to do that deliberately, and then directing it the way you want to direct it, is what hypnosis is all about.

Understood in this context, then, one does not have to be fearful of hypnosis. No one can (or is going to) take control away from you: you are going to learn how to have more control over *yourself*. I believe that finding out more about what we really think, and need, and want, and feel, instead of what other people think we should think, or need, or want, or feel, gives us far *more* control than we might otherwise have.

Is it possible for some unscrupulous person to take advantage of a psychologically vulnerable patient under the guise of "hypnosis"?

Of course it is. It's also possible for some unscrupulous person to take such advantage in a myriad of other ways, no less abhorrent.

Hypnosis is a tool which you learn, and then adapt and use for yourself. It's nice to have some guidance from a professional, but the one who uses the hypnosis is the patient, not the therapist. The talent for hypnosis comes from within YOU—part of your own rich inner pool of strengths and resources.

I made a brief reference to hypnotic pain relief techniques at the end of Chapter Two. Let's expand on them now.

We've discussed *relaxation* fairly thoroughly already. In altered states of consciousness, remember (I've read somewhere that people have to be exposed to an idea three times before it really clicks!) that there is a release of muscle tension, which is always accompanied by some improvement in comfort level. Tight tense muscles are more *un*comfortable than relaxed muscles.

The *dissociative* techniques are the quintessential hypnosis techniques because they layer a dissociative process on to a dissociative process. As mentioned in Chapter Two, there are two ways to use these: erect in your imagination some sort of barrier between yourself and the pain; or, put some distance between yourself and the pain.

I have had a cancer patient, who was coping well and didn't want to up her morphine, tell me that she would ". . . just leave my "painful body" on the bed while I went out and did the dishes." This is pure dissociation, of the putting-some-distance-in-between kind.

Women in the first stage of labor often use the distancing technique, going out to explore the galaxies (or whatever) and letting their bodies get on with the job; then, as the contraction ebbs, they come back into their bodies until the next one.

Descriptions of "floating above the pain," of "knowing it's there but it isn't part of ME," of "keeping it behind the barricade" all refer to dissociative techniques. Does one have to go into a formal hypnosis to do this? No—it's the other way around: by doing them, you take yourself into an altered state. Children will often imagine going off in a space ship (which of course is immune to any invasion by pain-aliens) or build tall imaginary walls to keep the pain out.

A useful hypnotic trick is to establish a code word to refer to whichever dissociative experience one has constructed; then, should the pain come on again and take one unawares, one may get faster relief by repeating (vigorously and often aloud) the code word. It is, of course, a post-hypnotic suggestion. Some people also use a code word to reinforce the relief.

Another type of dissociative technique has to do with time.

Earlier on, when Samantha was beginning to use her hypnosis effectively, I had asked her about the time *between* headaches.

"There IS no time between headaches," she stated positively. "The headache is there all the time. It's just that sometimes it isn't as bad as other times."

"Do me a favor," I begged her, "and keep track of the times between. Just for this week. It may surprise you."

She was clearly unimpressed with my suggestion but, being the good little patient that she was (can't afford to offend the new doctor), she agreed.

She came back the next week absolutely astounded. "I *do* have some times between headaches!" she said. "I didn't believe it when you said it, but I *do*!"

"Great," I responded, secretly thanking my lucky stars that this ploy had worked, "that gives us a whole new approach."

"What's that?"

"You're good at hypnosis," I told her. She nodded. "In hypnosis, as you know, time gets distorted." She nodded again. "Use your hypnotic talent," I said, mentally crossing all my fingers and toes as I made the suggestion, "to make the time *between* the headaches seem longer."

She looked at me dubiously, then smiled. This was a new challenge! She nodded. "I'll tr—," she started to use the word 'try', which she knew was a no-no in my office.* "I'll *explore the possibilities*!" she said triumphantly.

"Great," I responded. "I'm sure you can do it."

She could, and she did. She was shifting the emphasis *away* from the pain, *toward* the more comfortable interludes and, in so doing, was gradually regaining the sense of controlling

---

*We often underestimate the impact of language. For example, my patients know that the word 'try' is a no-no in my office; implicit in the definition of that word, is the possibility of failure, and so I say "search, learn more about, explore (a particularly good substitute) but please, *stop trying*! I'll talk more about the impact of language in Chapter Seven.

her life, which had been missing over the previous several years.

The technique of changing one's experience of time is really plagiarized from a Swedish friend who told me about it. It seemed like a wonderful idea, and I have used it successfully in a variety of situations. One can make distressing time seem shorter, or comfortable time seem longer, or the time *between* seem longer or shorter, whichever suits best.

Distraction is an alternate form of dissociation, one that children particularly enjoy. There is an exceptional video, available through the Canadian Cancer Society in Vancouver, called "No Fears, No Tears: Children with Cancer Coping with Pain." It was produced by a Vancouver psychologist, Dr. Leora Kuttner, at Children's Hospital in Vancouver. In it, several of the distraction techniques are demonstrated by children actually using them to keep comfortable during painful procedures. It's an emotional video—keep the kleenex handy—and quite wonderful.

Many chronic pain patients have discovered for themselves the merits of distraction. I believe that many of them have developed a "distraction ego state"—one that comes and takes over in those situations. This ego state is able to push the pain-ridden self away for periods of time while s/he (the ego state) indulges in whatever form the distraction takes—enjoying a book, listening to music, even writing a term paper or something equally absorbing and demanding.

The *substitution* techniques are slightly different. When using these, one deliberately substitutes one factor for another to change the scenario—to change the choreography, in fact.

Of course, there are spontaneous substitution situations, as we mentioned in Chapter Two. These examples just serve to emphasize the *normalcy* of these techniques. They're not strange or cloaked in mystery or dangerous to the soul—they're *normal* ways of coping with various circumstances, adapted into usefulness in the chronic pain arena. Experiencing a different *place* for the pain, a different *time* for the pain, or a different *feeling* for the pain can make a huge difference when pain is a constant companion, all the time, every day.

Let's say Mildred had to present at a staff meeting. She knew her stuff, but she was really afraid that her chronic neck pain would overtake her. Mildred might have coped with this possibility by doing some *contracting* around the issue of time—such as saying to herself (making a contract between ego states) "I need to have a clear head for this presentation. I'm going to ask my subconscious to help give me a couple of clear hours, free from this wretched, permeating neck pain, so that I can do this job well." The "contract" with the subconscious is for "a couple of clear hours" and that may very well be what Mildred gets, with her neck really letting her know who's boss after the presentation is over. However, the contract for substituting a different *time* held firm, and she did a good job.

Impossible, you say? It's not, you know. You've probably used some variation of it yourself, unaware of what you were doing at the time. A woman of my acquaintance (me) took a very bad fall and tore the ligaments in her (my) ankle. It was an intense, throbbing pain. She (I) was due at a conference in a couple of days and had to get her workshop ready. The pain made any thinking difficult, so she deliberately changed the rhythm of the pain, from a throb, to a cacophony, to rock 'n roll, to Mozart. (She loves Mozart but does not relate to cacophony!) Later, she and I (different ego states) went to the hospital for x-rays, etc., and got it bound up properly.

I will admit that this may be easier to do in the acute, rather than the chronic, pain situation. But if it works in one—hey! why not find out how it works for the other?

An extension of these techniques is to *change the image of the pain*. First, as we've said, one must find out what the image of the pain is. This may involve confering with various ego states, as some of them may experience it differently. This makes sense within our metaphor—that one's life becomes choreographed around the pain, and the dancers—inside and out—perform the dance routines according to their particular roles.

There is almost always one part of the self which is completely involved with the pain. That is frequently the part which *takes over* in the chronic pain situation. That part of the self will have a different image of the pain than, for instance, that part of Mildred which pushed it aside in order to make her presentation.

If you experience pain, especially chronic pain, take a little time to find out what the image of *your* pain is. Does it have a size, a shape, an edge, a thickness, a consistency? What color is it? (Pain almost always has a color.) What temperature—e.g., icy, burning, red-hot? Some people image their pain as an animal or a monster or a cartoon-like character. I've heard it described as a boa constrictor, and as a gnawing rodent.

A few years ago, I was privileged to participate for a day in a multidisciplinary pain clinic in Sweden, run by an anaesthesiologist colleague, Dr. Basil Finer. During part of the day, I looked at some of the paintings which had been done by the patients during the course of their in-patient time at the clinic.

The paintings expressed, in vivid form and color, the experience of their pain. One set in particular grabbed my attention. Upon entering the clinic, one patient's painting was of a sweet border of small flowers, like the edging one sometimes sees on personal note paper. As the weeks passed, and she got in touch with her feelings of anxiety, guilt, sorrow, and the flood of rage which she finally allowed to express itself, the paintings displayed dramatic change. One would not have thought they could have come from the same person. In fact, in a way, they didn't—because those parts of herself which had been denied a voice finally rose up and shrieked out their agony in vicious form and vibrant color. Recognition conferred validity, and with that, easing of the intense pain began.

One patient described her headaches as "an icicle stabbing deep into my eye"; descriptions of pain as a "vise-like grip" are common; a woman with cancer said it was like "a bear eating away at my intestines." Once the image has been expressed—in words, in paint, in sound (one patient composes music to express his feelings)—change is happening.

Other hypnotic techniques such as the glove anaesthesia, the participant observer ("That's me down there having pain, but I'm just going to stay away because that way, I don't have to feel it"), changing the intensity of the pain on some sort of measuring device, or giving it a name and talking to it in a friendly manner—all can be explored. If all else fails (but only failing for the time being), ask the subconscious mind what IT would do to ease the dolor that is always there with chronic pain. You may get a remarkable response from this conversation with yourself.

4. Other Techniques

Just a reminder again about techniques such as acupuncture and acupressure, Reiki or perhaps even reflexology. Many people have had a great deal of benefit from such approaches.

I confess that I don't understand how some of these approaches, such as reflexology, work; but if I've learned anything in twenty-five years in medicine, I've learned *not* to say that something's impossible just because I don't understand it. As long as it isn't harmful, or precludes other recognized therapy, I feel comfortable about it if it helps the patient to feel better.

Massage therapy is obviously very relaxing and comforting, especially to those with a fair amount of muscle tension incorporated into their pain.

Chiropractic and homeopathy offer other avenues to explore.

COPING SKILLS

Many coping skills have been mentioned in passing, but we'll gather some of them together here in a more cohesive form. Most of them come under the general heading of stress management techniques.

It will be of no surprise to anyone that learning how to diminish stress is an important aspect of relieving the *distress* of chronic pain.

Actually, when Dr. Hans Selye first described the Stress Response, he used the word 'stress' as the neutral interlude between the instigators—which he deemed 'distress' and 'eustress' [good stress]—and the result in the body. This is rather like using the word 'energy' as the neutral interlude between the sources of power which create energy—electric, hydro, nuclear, wind, solar, etc.—and the result to which that energy is put—lighting lights, turning windmills, heating houses and so on. But we have come to use the term 'stress' to be almost synonymous with *distress*. This is too bad, because stress is more often useful than not. We all need some challenge to make our lives more interesting and rewarding. It's when stress is negative, rather than positive, that we need to find different ways to manage it and, with a little luck, transform it into something positive. However, I will use the term in its commonly-accepted sense and you can just remember that in many cases, stress is very good indeed.

The stress response is an integral part of the pain response, again because of the biochemistry and outpouring of hormones which are involved. Some factor comes along sparking further demands which in turn create more stress. It behooves us, therefore, to include stress management in any chronic pain relief program.

1. Problem-Solving Techniques

Have you ever noticed how, when you are really 'stressed out' about something, small hurdles that would ordinarily not merit a moment's worry all of a sudden become huge mountains? Then, after the immediate difficult demand is dealt with, all of a sudden the mountain is back to being just a small hurdle again.

This is a fairly common experience, I'm sure. When you are in that state, however, and the 'problem' is looming large, and you're going around in circles because half of your mind is somewhere else, it really does help if you have some little gimmick up your sleeve just to break the cycle. The fact that you know it's a gimmick doesn't matter—you can laugh at yourself and think, "This is so silly!"—but if it works, don't knock it.

Most of the problem-solving techniques that work well are very simple; and most of them have some means of breaking the BIG problem down into small manageable pieces. Often they involve using one's imagination.

To demonstrate this, let's consider Nora, one of our fictional examples. Nora works in a demanding office where she is the head of her department, with a staff of six. Ordinarily, nothing much fazes her. Lately, however, there are problems at home with two teen-agers acting out (in different directions), a mother-in-law who needs a lot of attention, and rumors of job cuts at the plant where her husband works.

Nora usually copes with this concoction of challenges fairly smoothly, but lately she has been plagued with a return of persistent pain in one shoulder that dates back many years, but which had subsided somewhat until about six months ago. The pain makes her tense and snappy, which doesn't help with (a) her staff, (b) her teen-agers, (c) her mother-in-law, or (d) her husband.

One day the boss comes in and gives Nora's department yet another project to handle, and her staff rebel. "We can't do this," they say, angrily, "and get through all our other work, too."

What to do? Nora can feel the pain shooting across her shoulder as she wonders desperately how she, and her staff, are going to manage. Then she remembers a gimmick that she used to use when she was grappling with learning how to do this job, years ago. She calls her staff: strategy huddle!

"I think the only way to tackle this is in small pieces," she suggests. "What do you say?" They nod.

"When I was first learning this job, and I didn't know what to do next because there seemed to be so much of it, I used to use the alphabet."

The alphabet? They all look at her blankly.

"Yes, the alphabet. I'd start with the letter A and glance over my work load to see if there was something that began with A and, if there was, I'd do it. If there wasn't I'd go to B, and so on. It was just a silly gimmick, but it seemed to work. After a while, I would at least have done *something* and it didn't seem so overwhelming. Shall we see how it might work for us with this job?"

They agree, albeit somewhat reluctantly. Nora assigns each a letter in a round robin fashion and that person looks over the project to see what can be found that fits. Amazingly enough, with a little ingenuity, they all find something that "fits" and the project gets underway.

And (as Nora had hoped would happen), once they get started, their camaraderie surfaces and they spend the better part of an hour there, the six of them and Nora too, getting the first part of the project at least well-begun. Also, as the good feelings grow even warmer between them, Nora's shoulder doesn't bother her so much.

This is a gimmick. But, like all good gimmicks, all it really is, is a slightly different framework within which to describe the job at hand. Nora's shoulder naturally becomes more comfortable as the tension lets up both physically and emotionally.

Another problem-solving technique is *delegating*. Why do so many of us find it so hard to delegate? I think it has something to do with feeling *responsible* for things—for everything, in fact. But in reality, the ability to delegate wisely is a tremendous skill and is one of the things which identifies a good leader. I have suggested to people (not only to patients, but also to business groups in my seminars on stress management) that they *rehearse* delegating some task, within the safe cocoon of hypnosis. For example, they go into a comfortable level of self-hypnosis and imagine the situation in explicit detail, working out the delegating—what to whom—and then, speaking in a firm, business-like voice to the delegatee(s), remembering to give realistic time-frames within which to finish the task.

If you have a REAL problem with delegating, start with some *very, very small* task and gather strength from how well it's handled by the person to whom you delegate it. Remember, when delegating is done well, it reflects back very positively on you, the delegator—how you chose the right person, the right project, and the right time. Then you'll have a success in hand that will give you courage to tackle delegating something a tiny bit bigger!

So often, the "problem" in problem solving melts away when we give the whole thing a different definition. I ask my stress management groups: what is the definition of a problem? Most people answer "something that has to be coped with" or "a stumbling block" or "a difficult decision." I suggest that we define a problem as "an opportunity to do something different"—and that DOES give it a whole new connotation.

What to do differently? Anything! Assign it a new name. Change the order of the subsections, or divide it up differently, or change the dates by which some part of it must be finished. You can even *up* the date by which some (smaller) part of it must be finished and then bask in the glow of your progress. Most effective of all, ask your subconscious to help you shift your response to this "problem" and that will have already begun if you embrace the new definition. When we shift the response, we shift the weight of the burden—much the same as when we are carrying something very heavy, and we stop to shift the distribution of the weight, or adjust the straps on the backpack. We all know how that can make the load seem easier to carry.

Maybe the problem which is making your burden heavier and literally more painful has to do with family dynamics. These coping strategies work in those situations, too. Grit your teeth and give your teen-ager a responsible task, even if—no, *especially* if— said teen-ager has not been notable in the family for carrying out assigned tasks. Be sure that it is a legitimate task. Kids are able to sniff out a sop to their self-identity faster than you can say abracadabra and will give it the sneer it deserves. (Same goes for recalcitrant spouses.)

2. New Definitions

This really follows right along from what we were thinking about above. We could, for example, re-define the day; it doesn't have to have twenty-four hours, or even be separated into morning, afternoon, and night. Instead, it could be called 'more energy,' 'some energy,' and 'less energy'; or 'moving-about time,' 'slowing-down time,' and 'lying-down time'; or 'action time,' 'drag time,' and 'sleep time'—

you get the general idea. Redesign your daily planner into more manageable pieces with fancy titles that reflect the possibilities.

The more one is able to redefine a burdensome situation or experience into something that lightens it up, even a little bit, the easier it is to bear.

3. Time Out

One of the most crucial factors in stress management is to *take time for yourself*. Whether this is indulging in your favorite hobby, daydreaming, listening to music, going to the spa, meditating or self-hypnosing, having a long luxurious bath, working in your garden, reading or watching TV—whatever is right for you, be sure to take *some* time for yourself each day. If it's a very busy day and you only have five minutes, okay, take five minutes. But believe me, if you say that you don't have time to do this simple self-soothing, then I think it might be time to take a very hard look at your priorities. *Everybody* deserves at least five minutes of their own time, every day. And not when you're so tired that you'll fall asleep, either. This is a sometime-IN-the-day need. Prearrange it and schedule it right into your busy day. You'll get much more done, in the long run, when you fulfill this simple, basic need.

4. Activity

When we are under stress of any sort, the body is flooded with activity hormones and the subconscious/body collaboration makes the myriad biochemical adjustments which reflect this.

If we are going around with all these internal demands for action, it is obvious that the best way to re-establish a more comfortable equilibrium is to release some of the fight-or-flight preparedness. That means engaging in some kind of activity to use up all that adrenalin.

For people in chronic pain, this often seems like an insurmountable dilemma. However, when one works with the physiotherapist and medical support staff in figuring out how this can be accomplished, often there IS some solution. Exercising in water, for instance, can be helpful. Isometric exercises, which do not demand too much energy, may be another possibility. Re-define "action"—it needn't mean jogging two miles or lifting weights.

PERTINENT POINTS FROM CHAPTER SIX

The first step toward changing the dance of chronic pain is to **accept the concept.**

Change happens **slowly** and begins in small ways.

One first needs to identify the roles which other people, and one's own ego states, dance.

To begin change, look to see which roles it might be **easiest to modify.**

Gentle confrontation, although sometimes difficult, is often required.

Lifestyle changes occupy a major place in the list of opportunities for change.

Contracting, for example with one's doctors, offers possibilities.

Analgesic medication alone is **seldom useful** in relieving chronic pain.

There is a variety of pain relief techniques which can help to **alleviate the suffering** component: These include mechanical measures, relaxation and similar techniques, and hypnotic techniques which include dissociation, distraction, and changing the image of the pain.

Improving general **coping skills** is always helpful.

Stress management techniques include problem solving techniques, new definitions, and taking time out for oneself.

WORKSHEET FOR CHAPTER SIX

1. How and where can you start modifying the interaction between inside and outside "dancers"?

2. Make a list of potential modifications:

3. Which pain relief techniques appeal to you the most?

4. Which coping skills do you think would be most helpful for **you**?

5. What are some areas for lifestyle change in your particular situation?

6. How might you change any sabotaging family dynamics?

CHAPTER   SEVEN

ENDURING RELIEF

Further Changes

In Chapter Six, we looked at a variety of approaches and techniques which offered possibilities for "Changing The Dance." Let's carry on with that.

MORE COPING SKILLS

1. Getting Things in Order

I have a friend who, when she's sick and has to stay home in bed, will spend hours tidying up the bedroom so that she can relax enough to stay there. She just can't bear to be in the middle of a muddle when she's feeling lousy. The fact that the bedroom looks perfectly okay to anyone else is beside the point—she sees every book out of place on the shelves, every garment hung up sloppily, every dust ball in every corner.

People with chronic pain often despair at the disorder in their lives. Because there are so many things which they *cannot* seem to get in order, they may feel a great urgency to make things orderly whenever and wherever they can.

This makes sense. To focus on creating an orderly arrangement of things which one *can* control takes some of the sting out of not being able to control so many other intrusions into one's life. Remember, we have talked about chronic pain being an *intrusion*. The need to prevent disorder from also intruding is surely understandable.

Arranging things in an orderly fashion may mean, for instance, keeping a detailed daily planner; being meticulous about getting rid of clutter in the home; and considering *priorities*, which will be discussed in the next section. The important thing is to find the best way to do this so that the doing of it does not, itself, add to the intrusion.

2. Priorities

"I just don't know what to do next! And I'm in so much pain anyway—I don't feel like doing *anything* next!"

Sound familiar? I've heard it hundreds of times, and I'll bet you have, too, and perhaps have even said it once or twice yourself.

Sorting out priorities IS a priority for the chronic pain sufferer. When there is only so much time in the day when you feel able to tackle a few tasks, it is vital to know which of the myriad of things waiting in the wings (to get back to the dance metaphor!) are the most important for that particular time.

What we often forget, is that priorities change according to our circumstances and at different times in our lives. An interesting exercise is to take a piece of paper and a pencil and write down the top ten priorities in your life *today*. It's important to write them down just as they occur to you, without analyzing them and certainly without any judgement as to their "merit." For the purpose of this exercise, whatever occurs to you has equal merit. Then put the list away.

Some time later—I usually suggest six months, but that can certainly be debated—do the same thing: take a piece of paper and a pencil and write down the top ten priorities that come into your mind at *that* time, again in the order which they occur to you.

Compare the lists. I guarantee that they will be different. Some of the items on list number one will not be on list number two, and vice versa; and those that are on both lists will often occupy different places on the list. (If you are reading this book with the hope of finding ways to relieve your chronic pain, the idea of writing lists and comparing them six months from now will probably seem ludicrous. Just keep the *concept* in mind.) What's the moral of this story? Simply that our priorities change over time, in order to be consistent with whatever is taking precedence in our lives.

However, too often we then "try" to accommodate to ALL the priorities, both past and present. I call it being trapped by our old priorities. How can anybody fulfill such demands? The stress of attempting to do so is overwhelming and will certainly contribute to experiencing more pain.

Think about these "dance vignettes."

Matilda still goes to visit her mother twice every day in the Care Home because she has done that since her mother moved in there three years ago, and she feels very guilty if she misses even one of those visits. Now Matilda's husband, Tom, has an opportunity to go on a cruise, courtesy of his company, and he wants her to come with him (also courtesy of the company). "We never do anything together anymore," says Tom. "And when you get home from visiting your mother in the evening, your back hurts so much that all you can do is go and lie down. I think it would be good for you to go on this cruise, to relax and enjoy the sun, and I think it would be good for *us* too. Please come."

Daniel has coached the neighborhood little league in baseball for the past six seasons. He particularly enjoyed doing this because two of his sons were in the little league during that time. However, last winter his car was rear-ended and he sustained a miserable whiplash which still bothers him a great deal, despite neck braces and physiotherapy and medication and acupuncture and "you-name-it-I've-tried-it." He'd like to be able to just relax on weekends now, particularly since his sons are older and have gone on to other sports, but he feels that he has an obligation to the community to keep on coaching; so he has been doing that, and feeling very much out of sorts (he wouldn't like to use the word 'angry') as a result.

Joan and Jerry have been known as the neighborhood hosts for years. Not only do people from all over the country (and sometimes other countries) come to visit them and stay for days to weeks at a time, but all the neighbors drop in, too, for coffee or brunch or to shoot the breeze in the evening. It's just always been one of the things to do. And Joan and Jerry have two grown-up kids, both married, and five grandchildren who absolutely adore coming over to visit Grandma and Grandpa on the weekends. All this was okay when Joan and Jerry were younger, but now that they are well into their mid-seventies, they'd really love to have a little peace and quiet. Joan has arthritis, which gives her what-for a lot of the time, and Jerry gets awful lumbago. But they feel that they couldn't disappoint all those folks and it *is* so nice to see them. Still . . . .

All of these folks are trapped by their own **past** priorities. They need to take a good look at what they need for themselves at *this* time of their lives and make changes accordingly. Of course this does not mean stopping the visits to mother, or never coaching little league again, or putting a 'no guests' sign on their doors. It *does* mean taking a good look at today's priorities and going with those, for today. Tomorrow things may be different again.

Samantha and Dave had always had separate bank accounts and had shared household expenses equally through the many years they had been together. But Samantha, in her working days, was a much higher wage earner than Dave, so when 'extra' things came along, she was usually the one who paid for them.

That had seemed to work well for them, so when she came in, obviously furious, and started talking about household finances, I wondered what on earth had gone wrong.

There were a lot of aspects, but one was, of course, that she was now on a Disability Pension and did not have nearly the same income that she had been used to.

Apparently Dave, in a desperate attempt to save her any worry, had gotten himself in over his head and hadn't a clue as to how to tell her. Finally it had come to a crisis and the whole thing had come out.

She'd had some major headaches, too, and *that* hadn't helped.

In the long run (after some stormy sessions), this resulted in a serious re-evaluation of their priorities and their lifestyle, and a rearrangement of how they handled their financial affairs.

3. Language

We greatly underestimate the impact of language. Remember that people in pain, anxious, ill, or traumatized, are indeed in an altered state of consciousness and may very well misinterpret what they hear, hearing only a part of it, or ignoring a 'not,' for example.

What we also must remember is that these same premises apply when we are talking *to ourselves*.

Self-talk is going on all the time, inside our heads. Some part of our awareness (perhaps barely at the conscious level) is carrying on a constant running commentary, even when we are talking aloud, and even when we are listening intently to someone else. Many people call it "The Chatterbox." But it is most evident when we are daydreaming, or mulling over something, or wishing we had said something other than what we did say, or carrying on imaginary conversations in our minds that always go the right way because we can make the other party say what we *want* them to say so that we can respond with our next brilliant comment.

Unfortunately, we never do that kind of revised edition when we are talking to ourselves. Too bad, because so much of our self-talk is disparaging, contradictory, and/or sabotaging.

Just listen:

"I'm such a klutz—if I hadn't [done whatever] this would never have happened."

"I *always* do these stupid things!"

"I'll never get over this, never."

"No wonder my doctor gets fed up with me—I'm so miserable that [she or he] couldn't possibly care what happens to me."

"I'll never amount to anything, anyhow."

"My [mother, father] always told me that something terrible would happen if I didn't smarten up."

These internal dialogues promote *healing*? Of course not, how could they? They promote more pain—emotional and (because of tension) physical.

We all need to learn better strategies for positive self-talk. There's been a lot of discussion about ego states earlier in the book. Here's a chance for those ego states to get something going that's different.

Choose your ego state participants. Of course, this will make it seem even more artificial than it already does, but that's okay. Then, let your self-doubting or negative or tired-of-it-all ego state make some appropriate comment; and then have a positive part of yourself answer back, strongly and with vigour, refuting the negativism. Make it a game—things often work better that way, especially when we're just beginning to explore a whole new way of looking at things.

Learn to hear yourself when you say "try" or "should" and find out what that's all about. Why do you need to "try?" It implies the possibility of failure. If you're not sure about something, do like Samantha said and "explore the possibilities." And if you are saying "I should"—make sure you know where that "should" comes from: from you? from outside? Outside shoulds and inside shoulds often have entirely different agendas and that's why they clash.

Most important of all, learn to do affirmations. These are constant reminders to ourselves that we are striving toward a goal. They can be done at any time, whatever else we might be doing, in hypnosis or out of it, and in saying them we continuously remind ourselves of that goal. They also enhance self-esteem and self-image, rather than bruising the ego further by negative self-talk. An affirmation is a statement about the future, made in the present tense, as if it has already happened in the past (e.g., "It's wonderful to move more comfortably"). Therefore they imply that we are looking forward to success.

You can start to break out of the negative self-talk mold by taking all those 'downer' phrases and converting them, thus: "I'm such a klutz . . ." converts to "I move with balance and ease" or "I'll do it differently next time."

"I *always* do these stupid things" converts to "Another of life's lessons."

"I'll never get over this . . ." converts to "I'm looking forward to moving on with my life."

"No wonder my doctor . . ." converts to "My doctor and I can work together."

"I'll never amount to anything . . ." converts to "I will be the very best I can be" or the good old standby: "Every day in every way I'm getting better and better."

And as for "My [mother] always told me . . ."—reject that! Say, "I am proud of my achievements" or some such positive declaration.

What has all this to do with relieving chronic pain?

I believe that positive self-talk is central to deflecting the negative impact of day-in-day-out pain. By using positive self-talk we begin to change our mind-sets (in hypnosis jargon, we call it "creating a yes-set"). This change in mind-set is absolutely necessary for someone in chronic pain who is determined to get out of the pit of feeling like a victim.

It is a way of saying to the pain, "*I refuse to let you rule my life any longer. Although it will be one of the biggest challenges I have ever undertaken, I am going to shift this burden that has overwhelmed me for so long. I can do this, and I will do this. I know that pain may be my companion, now, but a companion is different from a tyrant. Goodbye, tyrant!*"

As change begins to creep in—a softening of impact here, a lightening of the burden there—be sure to say "Thank you" to yourself for these good things that you are doing. To do so adds great strength to your resolve; to forget to do so implies that it isn't very important anyway.

Another kind of language that packs a wallop is body language, and this turns up in self-talk all the time. There are two kinds of body language. One is demonstrated in posture, for instance, or facial expression. The other is implicit in the metaphors and similes with which we describe ourselves. The English language (and, I am sure, all other languages) is rife with these: how about "shouldering the task"; "putting your shoulder to the wheel"; being "backed against the wall"; needing to "stand on my own two feet"; it "makes me sick"; "my heart aches for you"; having the "weight of the world on your shoulders." (Remember how hard it is for some people to delegate? They are continuing to carry the

weight of the world on their shoulders!) And there's another connection here—what do you get when you detach the 'ers' from
'shoulders'? Um-hum—'*should.*' It's an interesting glimpse at the
way language can subconsciously affect us, isn't it?

When we deliberately change the language, we off-set these implications.

Ego-strengthening self-talk is so very important that it deserves
another paragraph.

Remembering to say "thank you" to ourselves is ego-strengthening. It strengthens the core self when we pay respectful and ap-
preciative acknowledgment to the work that we are doing for ourselves. With all the diverse ego states that blossom when we are
in pain, it is even more important to bolster the strong parts of
ourselves and help the overwhelmed parts to heal. Vigorous internal dialoguing can promote this shift toward the positive and
thus, perhaps slowly but also surely, toward relief from the ab-
solute intrusion of chronic pain.

Samantha and I began to explore the implications of her
feeling that, without her work, she was really nothing.

The most immediate concern was how this related to her
feeling that she was to blame for her headaches, that if only
she could somehow be a better person, the headaches would
go away.

Since being a better person was inextricably linked to her
professional, working persona, in Samantha's mind, if she
couldn't work then, by perverse logic, neither could she be
a worthwhile person and—ergo—would never be able to get
away from the headaches.

There was no point in being cognitive about this. She recognized that her self-doubts were rooted deep and long and
were essentially emotional. "It's pretty hard to change an
emotional response through a logical process," I told her,
and she agreed.

One day she arrived at the office, arms laden with loose-
leaf binders, crammed to the limit. They were some of the
diaries that she had kept from high school days. She was
quite excited.

"I can see it all beginning, right in these pages," she said.
"They're all really letters to myself—I even sign them that
way."

"Yes, you have. What do you suppose that means?"

"I think I was searching for myself, not sure of who I was even then."

"That's pretty common for teen-agers," I commented.

"Yes, but this is different. When I was a teen, I was often a miserable, rebellious kid. I think it was my way of finding some sort of strength—strength that I was afraid wasn't really there. I think I carried that right through into my adulthood. Work gave me someone to be, and so it *became me.*"

"And now?"

"I guess I have to start finding out about myself, who I am, all over again."

"But this time, you understand much more about what you're doing," I offered.

"Yes. But somehow I don't think that's going to make it very much easier."

COGNITIVE CHANGES

Of particular interest, when we are thinking of cognitive changes, are the comments of Dr. Basil Finer, which are reported in the section on research in Chapter Nine.

He remarks on the pain patient's *different reality*—a reality built around pain; pain supports this reality, pervades it, encompasses it. The patient's life *is* pain. In order to alter this reality, one must gain access to it.

Obviously that means, as a baseline, that the doctor or therapist can assure the patient that even though there is no apparent "reason" why the patient has this pain, nevertheless there is no question that the pain is real. Following from that, the sufferer often needs to be repeatedly assured that no serious organic illness has been missed.

These two needs seem to be poles apart, and actually contradictory, from the patient's view—if it's real, then how can anybody know that there isn't something seriously wrong? Part of the cognitive work is to explain what appropriate investigation entails, and at what point it becomes counterproductive to continue to search for answers that are not—at least at this stage of our knowledge—available to us.

(How enticing, though, the idea that perhaps the pain patient is somehow neurologically supersensitive to pain, as Dr. Helen Crawford suggests in one of her papers, and that anyone who has those supersensitive neural pathways is a potential chronic pain patient.)

Cognitive approaches may take many forms. They could mean, for instance, exploring *pain behavior* with the patient. This might involve the keeping of diaries, monitoring sleep patterns, discussing and attending to changing dietary needs, or recognizing the fatigue potential of various activities including interaction with other people—family and non-family.

Specific techniques within the cognitive framework include behavior modification, which of course fits right in with exploring the unique pain behavior of a particular person. Behavior modification will also include physio- and occupational therapy, and a specific rehabilitation program usually aimed toward getting the patient back to work.

This latter goal is often an emotional mine-field for the patient, who longs to be able to go back to work but is deadly afraid of being forced back when he or she cannot do the job. Those realities must also be explored from a cognitive perspective.

Constructing useful contracts (as mentioned earlier) is another cognitive opportunity. It is always interesting to record changes in attitude—by both the professional and the client/patient—when such contracting is done.

To illustrate this, let's consider another combined case.

Harriet was an astute businesswoman and a well-known speaker in her field. She had strong opinions with a wealth of properly researched factual information. All in all, some folks found her a bit overwhelming but no one denied her capability.

As she neared her fortieth birthday, Harriet began to experience a lot of vague pain throughout her body. It seemed to migrate around. Her doctor told her it was probably rheumatism, which offended her. In the first place, there was no history of rheumatic disease of any sort in her family and secondly, it made her sound old and feeble.

Harriet had had a tough life, with an alcoholic father and an ineffectual mother. She had had to be a surrogate parent to her younger brother and sister from the time she was just a child herself. She had fulfilled that role, and was still fiercely protective of her siblings even though both were adults and leading their own lives (not too well, in her opinion, but by that time they weren't consulting her).

As the next few months passed, the pain began to localize more and she recalled that she had read somewhere about something called fibromyalgia. She went to her family doctor, insisting that she be referred to Dr. X, a specialist in rheumatology who was known to be familiar with this disorder. After carrying out a thorough investigation, including blood tests, x-rays, and a muscle biopsy, Dr. X told her that, in his opinion, she did indeed suffer from fibromyalgia. He also told her, bluntly, that she was going to have to modify her lifestyle.

Over the next few months, all of Harriet's aplomb and vigour seemed to melt away. She turned down speaking engagements and began to carry out her job in a perfunctory manner that was quite unlike her. The pain intensified; her social life became almost non-existent. She was not married, nor in a committed relationship, and she seemed to have no interest in anything. Even her sister and brother started to get worried about her.

During this time she also began to make frequent appointments with her family doctor, exhorting him to *do* something. It became a battleground. She kept demanding that he consult again with Dr. X in order to get more insight.

Whether he ever did that, she never knew. But one day, when she went in to see him, he said to her, "Sit down in that chair there—" (indicating a chair with a small writing table beside it) "—and we are going to draw up some contracts."

And they did. They contracted around telephone calls, length and frequency of appointments, what to do in an emergency ("Ask yourself whether *I* will think it's an emergency," he said somewhat grimly), what medications she could expect him to prescribe and how frequently she could renew them, and Harriet attending aquacize sessions, led by a physiotherapist, at the local community center.

That session was hard on both of them, but at the close of it he offered his hand in a gesture of partnership and reconciliation. She took it.

In subsequent biweekly appointments of fifteen minutes each, they explored many cognitive issues, including her family background and her attitude to pain. She began to argue vigorously with him over various opinions regarding fibromyalgia (a good sign, he thought, but wearying!). They discussed interferences with sleep and how these contributed to pain—an aspect which she found fascinating.

Best of all, over the next several weeks they developed a new respect for each other. No longer were they antagonists: rather, they were partners.

This vignette illustrates several things, including the imperative that the patient is a *participating* dancer in this company, and that the doctor has to remember to be sensitively cognitive, too.

(In psychological jargon, these are transference and counter-transference issues which need to be recognized, because they can divert caregivers and therapists from our main objective, which is to relieve suffering and help the sufferer to resume an improved quality of life.)

REGAINING CONTROL

Someone once defined chronic pain patients as people who *used* to be in control of their lives.

It's a dismal definition.

The sense of being out of control of one's life is one of the most difficult aspects of any chronic illness. Furthermore, because so often people with chronic illnesses (fatigue, pain, some kinds of depression) appear to be so healthy, people "on the outside" have a hard time understanding why this otherwise intelligent being doesn't just pull up his or her socks and get back in the real world again. They don't understand that the fatigue, the pain, the depression have now *become* "the real world" for these patients.

Beginning to regain control is fraught with obstacles. Vulnerability, lack of information or understanding that information, fatigue, that miserable sense of dependency, fear (especially the "what if . . ." train of thought) and the distorted reality of constant pain all conspire to prevent sufferers from shifting the balance of power, between their inside and outside worlds and also between the positive and negative parts of themselves, back onto at least a half-way even keel.

Therefore, regaining control begins with a change in attitude, from the desperation of "I can't do anything about this" to "I will find some way to start doing something about this."

An *attitude* is usually *a response to a belief system*. To encourage our attitude to change, we must think about how to change the belief system:

Away From	*Toward*
desperation	determination
vulnerability	strength
feeling submerged	resurfacing
pain reality	open reality
I can't	I can
the pain is my life	I have a life and I also have pain
managing the pain	managing the comfort
	(courtesy of Samantha)

All very well, but how to get started?

1. Be Assertive

If necessary, take an assertiveness training course. (They're fun, and you can learn a lot about yourself—and about other people too.) Being assertive is entirely different from being aggressive, which only puts people's backs up. On the other hand, being mousy almost always results in feeling trapped. True assertiveness lies in the ability to state clearly and succinctly what and how you feel, and what and how you want to change. Almost everyone responds positively to quiet assertiveness, and I can pretty well guarantee that will include your doctor, too. Explain what you need—more information, a support group, a counselor, more time to express your fears—and negotiate around that. Which brings us to—

2. Negotiate

True negotiation involves listening carefully to the concerns of the other side, and reaching workable agreements. Sometimes just listening carefully and making a response such as "I'm beginning to understand your perspective" can get everything rolling. For one thing, it disarms the opposition! (Fellow doctors, take note.)

3. Promote Openness

When we are open and frank with our thoughts and feelings (obviously avoiding put-downs and the poor-me syndrome), it encourages a similar openness from those with whom we are communicating. This goes for family, friends, doctors, disability evaluators, and the family pet. ("I'm sorry, Henrietta, but you can't curl up and go to sleep on my lap because I have to be able to move frequently in order to be more comfortable. But I'll put a nice soft blanket in your basket.")

Whimsy aside, it does feel better to be able to say what you need to say. Having to avoid certain topics makes for stultifying conversation. Be prepared, however, for your assertive listener to state openly that s/he doesn't want to hear any more [about your condition]!

This happened to a patient of mine. Lillian had had a horrid Bell's palsy and was still in misery with her post-viral pain almost two years after the viral infection itself had resolved. She and I had been discussing these controlling-your-life issues and she came in one day, gave me an accusing eye, and said, "Well, I've been doing what you told me." [Whoops!] "I've been talking openly and assertively and making my needs understood. And do you know what happened to me yesterday? One of my very best friends told me in no uncertain terms that he now knew more than he had ever wanted to know about post-herpetic neuralgia!"

4. Make Decisions

Awful things happen to people who are conquered by chronic pain. Among other disastrous possibilities, they often lose the ability to make even normal day-to-day decisions. This is, of course, utterly demoralizing. "I can't even decide whether to wear my grey sweats or my green cut-offs" or "You'd think it would be easy to decide what cereal to have for breakfast but somehow—" or "Even the *thought* of planning dinner overwhelms me" or "Jimmy asked me to make some cookies for his class party. I sat looking at my recipe book for two hours and still didn't know which ones to make" are the sort of wails that I hear from chronic pain sufferers who are grappling with decision making.

Well, these are good places to start. If you can't decide which clothes to wear, put both names in a hat and draw one out. (You will have decided to put the names in a hat.) To get Jimmy's cookies in the oven, shut your eyes and stick a pin somewhere in on the cookie list in the table of contents. (Yes, you decided to stick a pin.) In time—trust me if you can—you'll get tired of making choices in this way and will actually decide on some course of action.

Once you are back into the decision-making mode, you can extend your new (recovered—it was there all the time) ability to more important issues. Then you can participate in the decision-making process with regard to your rehabilitation plan. Which brings us to—

5. Participate

You *must* become a participant if you are ever going to feel like a normally intelligent human being again. Don't expect your doctor to drag you into participating—probably s/he hasn't time to do that and anyway, what would you gain? You're moving into independence, right? Right. Then participate independently. (In other words, recognize that you're a lead dancer.)

6. Reassess Frequently

As you learn more about where and how you can regain control, reassess the situation in light of new understandings—of yourself, of others, of the role of pain in people's lives. Remember that often, when you are talking with people, you have pain and they don't. Incorporate that into your assessment of the situation. It's no use expecting them to know how you feel. Nobody knows how you feel except you, or how I feel except me. We can be understanding, we can be sympathetic, we may even be able to use our imaginations to a certain extent, but the one person in the world who knows how you *really* feel, is you.

You know all this. In fact, you've probably even said a version of it in a different way—"How can you say that/think that/imply that/suggest that when you have no idea of what I'm *feeling*?!"

Understanding that 'no, that other person truly does *not* know what your pain feels like' will put things into a slightly different perspective. So pay attention to what people are telling you, while recognizing this one important fact: you have pain, and they don't.

7. Construct a WIB

A what? A WIB—a What-If Box. Almost everybody falls into the what-if trap from time to time. We're worried or anxious about something; we can think of all kinds of disastrous outcomes of situations; we wonder how or if we can cope. Generally those in-securities pass, but some people are expert what-if-ers, and have perfected it to a fine art. When one lives with chronic pain, this is an all-too-easy trap to fall into. There is no room for what-ifs when one is re-establishing control of one's life. Therefore—we need a gimmick. (Remember gimmicks in the problem-solving section? Great things, gimmicks.)

If you are talented at what-iffing, you will surely be talented at constructing a WIB, because both of those activities involve using one's powers of imagination. What-iffing, however, is using that power negatively whereas constructing a WIB is using it positively.

In your imagination, then, create the perfect WIB—the right size, shape, material, color—just right for you. Be sure that there is a one-way letter slot going *into* the WIB, which closes so that nothing can come back out. Also make sure it has an escape valve for the hot air that the what-if becomes, after the threat of its oc-curring has passed.

Then, whenever you hear yourself saying "what if"—consign it immediately to the WIB, where it can be guarded and taken care of properly.

The point is, in the chronic pain world, you're not dealing with *what if*; you're dealing with *what IS*. Clarifying those diverse in-terpretations will carry you a long way back into resuming con-trol of your life.

8. Deal with Saboteurs

There's been a lot of talk in earlier chapters about inside and out-side saboteurs. Dealing with the saboteurs is an essential part of the process of resuming control.

The most useful approach, I think, is to sort them out and give them something better to do. This may be more practical for the internal saboteurs than for those on the outside, but with a little ingenuity it can work for both. It's easier, of course, if the person in mind is also a helper—directing them towards new areas is usu-ally met with compliance and often with appreciation. This may not be so for any outside saboteurs who are really into undermin-ing you. (Question: *Why* would they want to undermine you? There's some negative dynamic going on here—as was the case with sisters Lois and Jackie—that needs exploring. In doing so, you may even find some opportunity to transform them into helpers.)

Internal saboteurs are more available to you. Just look back over your list of inside dancers—an honest appraisal, now—and see where there can be some shift. Remember the old adage that, if you want to defuse some antagonist's complaints, put him or her in charge of whatever s/he is complaining about? Works well! Adapt the same concept to your agitating ego states.

> Ellen's whole system was infused with anxiety over whether she should apply for a part-time job at the library. She had been a *good* librarian, she reminded herself, be-fore It Happened. Her doctors and her psychotherapist were all telling her that it would be good for her to get back into some part-time work again, and she'd made the mistake (as she thought now) of telling her therapist about this part-time job at the local branch.
>
> Fourteen months before, Ellen had been assaulted on her way home from work one evening. She had not been raped, but two ribs were broken and she'd had a concus-sion from a vicious blow to her head. Her injuries had healed, but she re-lived that assault over and over again. Her doctor sent her to a therapist who understood about posttraumatic stress disorder and she was slowly getting her life back in order, but so far none of that had helped the chest-wall pain which came upon her out of the blue and would last for hours.

Understanding about her ego states had, in fact, been part of her psychotherapy and it did make sense to her. She knew that there was a part of her which was terrified of getting assaulted again. But there was also a part of her which blamed herself, constantly, for getting mugged in the first place, and which said to her, "No wonder you have pain. Serves you right!"

This ego state was her main saboteur. As long as she felt that she deserved the pain, the suffering, she knew that it would be next to impossible to even ease it, let alone get rid of it.

With the help of her therapist, she explored what the sabotage was all about. She came to understand that, in a funny way, this part of her wanted to protect her from further harm, and figured that if she were scared out of her skin that she might be attacked again, she would never let herself get into such a vulnerable situation.

The breakthrough came when she spoke to that part of herself directly and asked it for some different kind of protection. To her astonishment, the ego state apparently complied, because her anxiety let up and, with it, the pain let up too. The apparent solution seemed too simplistic to be taken seriously: *Take a taxi home.* She applied for and got the part-time job, and she found herself, bemused, at the telephone after each shift, phoning for a taxi. This carried on long after she felt confident that she could handle the bus trip. She laughed about it, saying "The Old Cuss is still there, taking care of me, I guess."

9. Manage the Comfort Instead of the Pain

This means making the most of the comparatively comfortable times, and requires a shift in thinking. When you have chronic pain, and the pain pervades your life, it is natural to think in terms of "managing the pain." This was obvious with Samantha.

We had been working away at sorting out Samantha's outside and inside dancers, and her insight was growing every day. There was still no question in her mind about the Choreographer. "It's The Pain," she still stated positively.

She had also been working very hard on cognitive issues,

organizing her day so as to make the most of the best time. Ever since she had recognized that there *was* some time between headaches, her whole attitude changed.

But there was one phrase which she used time and again: *"managing the pain."* She spoke about how much energy it took to manage the pain; about how the medication managed the pain; about how so much of her day was spent managing the pain.

Feeling snarky myself one day, I said to her, "Do you think you could start managing the *comfort*?"

She looked at me blankly. "What do you mean?"

"You spend a lot of time talking about managing the *pain*," I said. "Could you shift that emphasis and start managing the *comfort* instead?"

This was obviously a whole new way of looking at things, and Samantha was good about those opportunities, willing to explore them. She sat back in the chair with a little thump. "That's a good question," she said. (This is a favorite phrase of hers.)

"Um-hum. So, how about it?"

"I'll work on it," she promised.

Managing the comfort instead of managing the pain illustrates, again, the importance of language. When you say those two different phrases, the whole connotation is different, and so is the response—the response by others who hear the words and, far more importantly, the response within the person who says them. Obviously the emphasis moves from pain to comfort and with that, the choreography changes too. No longer does the whole day revolve and dance around the *pain*. Some of the day, at least, begins to revolve and dance around the comfort.

10. Become the Lead Dancer

As these changes begin to evolve more definitively so will the roles of the ego states, and so will the roles of the outside dancers change in relationship to those changed internal dancers. The goal of the "host," therefore, (the host is the ego state which epitomized the person's personality *before* the chronic pain syndrome) is to once again become the lead dancer.

As more and more of the emphasis edges away from being subsumed by the pain, so also the choreography will also change. Luckily, this is inevitable.

The time for the host to reassert her/himself gets closer and closer and, as it nears, it is appropriate for some rehearsal of this new evolving dance to begin.

Tentatively, in my experience, the host begins to reorganize things—time, activities, priorities—always starting with something small and unthreatening. As little victories (no matter how small) appear on the stage, ego strength returns. Oh, it is fragile, and easily battened down again, so it takes diligence and perseverence. Jill has had three good nights' sleep so she plans to stay up a little later again to watch a favorite TV show. Just as she's settling down, she gets a dreadful spasm and some internal saboteur grabs the opportunity to say, "See? I told you you're not ready for anything like that!" as she staggers off to bed in agony. Jill's obvious inclination at that point is to vow never to stay up to watch a late TV show again in her whole life.

If one possibility doesn't work out, explore a different one. Gradually, things *do* begin to change and, as they do, so do the roles in The Dance. As these changes evolve, a new Choreographer emerges, directing this strong dance team. One might even postulate that the growing sense of self-esteem becomes the new Choreographer.

EMOTIONAL CHANGES

Emotions will be on a roller-coaster as the choreography slowly changes more and more, bit by bit.

Emotions are wonderful things. They bring color to our lives. Just let yourself imagine what it would be like to be bereft of emotional response—no joy, no wonderment, no resolve, no contentment, no despair, no anger, no jealousy, no guilt, no hope, no love.

"But," you protest, "I could cheerfully do without *some* of those emotions!"

Ah, yes. But without the negative emotions, we are cut off from all the positive ones too. Being capable of vibrant emotional response is kind of a package deal. You take the ones you like, you get the ones you don't like along with them.

As people become aware of their individual emotional responses, they can also begin to channel them into more comfortable harbors. A harbor is a place for keeping things safe. It's useful to find safe harbors for those emotions which overwhelm us, until we get ourselves reorganized a bit. It's like waiting in the wings, out of sight, until it's time to dance back on stage.

As the intrusion of chronic pain ebbs, the resurfacing patient finds that there are new demands upon him or her. People begin to *expect* something of them again. How about getting back into social life? Do you *still* need someone to do your shopping? Why can't *you* read the kids their bedtime story?

These expectations can be *very* scary. Samantha has pointed out that, if pain has been part of your life for ages, 'getting rid of it' quickly leaves too big a hole. We need to fill the hole, gradually, with healthier components.

Also, as the intrusion begins to ebb, hope emerges. Should it be temporarily dashed again, that can be very hard to take.

Expecting wild emotional rides helps to keep these emotions in perspective. It is also very useful to talk about them openly, preferably with a counselor. A friend's sympathetic ear may be comforting, but that friend may be too close to offer much in the way of objective feedback. However, if there is no counselor on the stage, by all means do a head hunt through the outside dancers and find one or two that would be most helpful. (Note: a person can be most helpful by responding with phrases like "Ummm," in a truly caring way.)

You can channel emotions through stating them clearly and then taking a careful look at what you said and, if necessary, deliberately rephrasing it.

> EXAMPLE: "I'll never get through this depression" might become, "This is a dark time. I'll be glad when it's over."
> EXAMPLE: "I cannot see beyond the pain" might become "I cannot see beyond the pain at this time."
> EXAMPLE: "My emotions are all over the place—it's terrible!" might become, "This emotional roller-coaster is certainly a challenge."

(If it is becoming even more evident that emotions and language are intertwined and that our language is emotionally laden and emotionally driven—you are right.)

There is a reason for examining emotions and redirecting them. When we are flooded with negative emotion, the physiological response is also very negative. Pain is exacerbated. Tension mounts. Sleep evades us.

On the other hand, when we neutralize that toxic negativism, and some positive response begins to creep in, the body responds positively—pain is less of an intrusion, we sleep better, we can make decisions. Read the work of Dr. Candace Pert. These are the sorts of things she was talking about. "Emotion is expressed in the body through neuropeptides," she says. And we can say, "Emotion is expressed by MY body through physical awareness, response, and sensation."

Ivan would pound out his anger on the table. This served a dual purpose, he felt—it let off some of the steam, and the consequent pain in his hand became a welcome distraction from the constant impression of knives tearing at the muscles between his shoulder blades. Believing that this was useful, he made no attempt to stop the behavior.

The angry outbursts frightened his wife, who was ordinarily what one of my colleagues calls a chameleon: she would become indistinguishable from the furniture or the wallpaper or (said with irony) the mat on the floor. Besides, the rages reminded her of her alcoholic father, which was a frightening thing for her.

It took tremendous resolve for her to confront Ivan about his fist-banging. At first he sneered at her, made derogatory remarks, and then gave her the cold shoulder treatment. She literally would take two or three very deep breaths and softly—but with growing emphasis—repeat what she had said.

This was new behavior for her (*she* was changing the dance!) and Ivan finally recognized the implications of this.

"What would you have me *do?*" he demanded. "Go crazy? Because that's what I feel is happening—I'm going crazy. And when I pound the table, I feel less crazy, more in control of myself—it's **me** that's pounding the table."

"But you think it brings you some relief, and it *doesn't*," she insisted. "It's just a smokescreen, that's what it is. Afterwards you feel just as bad as ever, and I think—" she gulped before going on "—I think that it even makes you feel a little guilty because you know it upsets me."

This was so close to the truth that Ivan was suddenly completely deflated.

"What do you think I should do?" he asked again, but in a different voice.

She gulped again. This was quicksand. "Well, I've read about those workshops out at the college—they call them anger workshops. I think there are people there who know about anger—what it does to people. Maybe they could help you."

He was speechless. Then he scoffed; he spouted sarcasm for a half-hour; he pointed out that nobody was going to tell *him* how to behave. But in the long run, when she held her ground with quiet stubbornness, he went.

She hardly dared believe her eyes and ears when he came home after those sessions. He was *changed*; he was a *changed man*. She wondered if the changes could possibly last.

Months later, she dared to bring the subject up. The workshops had led seamlessly into sessions with one of the counselors. Ivan almost never talked about what went on during those appointments. Finally she said, "Please don't think I want you to tell me anything that you don't want to talk about. But it seems to me that things are a little bit better for you—as if the pain doesn't bother you quite so much."

"I still have the knives in my back, all the time," he answered. "I guess the difference is that I don't twist them so much."

Ivan's story illustrates the importance of confronting the *anger* which inhabits all chronic pain patients. Some of these angry cauldrons are relatively easy to reach, while others are very deep indeed. Generally the anger is more deeply embedded when there is a subconscious perception that it somehow needs to be protected. Maybe it is too risky to acknowledge it. Maybe the person is afraid of what he or she might do, were the rage to be unleashed.

Understanding the roots of anger (these have already been cited as frustration, fear, intrusion and injustice) helps us to realize that there may be several ego state dancers who are in some way associated with these varying emotions—'frustration-anger' is not in the same ballpark as 'injustice-anger.'

Usually, assertive confrontation—in other words, telling how you feel to whomever it is necessary to tell—will deal quite well with the anger from frustration and also from fear (although there is often fear in the telling) and then people can take a couple of deep breaths and carry on. There won't be any miraculous change, but a bit of the burden will be lifted and the outside dancers cope surprisingly well with this. Honest!

The rage from intrusion and injustice is the kind that almost always needs some professional help. Going after this help is a sign of *strength*, not of weakness. Learning ways to bring the anger out into the daylight, safely, is infinitely better than allowing it to continue to erode one's very soul.

Dealing with the anger is an essential part of resuming control of your life.

S amantha came in looking stricken.
  "What on earth?" I asked. I hadn't seen her look like that before, not even when Dave had left for a while.

"Jessica [her G.P.—not her real name] got a letter from the College," she said, referring to the College of Physicians and Surgeons, the provincial monitoring body for all doctors. "They're coming down on her hard for all the medication she's been prescribing for me."

"But I thought your neurologist was prescribing it," I said.

"He's the one who keeps track of it and makes suggestions, but Jessica actually prescribes it."

"Ah. I see." This is a common way of doing things—it has the advantage of keeping all prescription drugs in one chart. "Have you spoken to him?"

"I have an appointment on Monday. I think he's had letters, too."

"Well, you can't do anything more right now. I'm sure Jessica is in touch with him, too."

"The worst thing," she burst out, "is what they said about me—that I'm not getting any better. And I've been doing *so much better!*"

She had a copy of the letter which stated, in part, that there was "no clinical improvement." This made me angry, too, because it was written by someone who had never set eyes on Samantha. The fact was, there was no *pharmaceuti-*

cal improvement—that is, she still consumed a lot of analgesics each day.

However, Samantha had reason to be so infuriated, because there *had* been a huge *clinical* improvement—that was what we had been focusing on.

She was also feeling guilty on behalf of her G.P. "Jessica can take care of herself," I said. "You concentrate on you."

It was months before this was resolved. Her neurologist had suggested submitting an application to have her condition classified as "Intractable benign pain syndrome," and this is what eventually happened. In connection with that, Samantha's medication was changed (to a more potent drug, ironically); she had a severe reaction to that; it was changed again—all in all, a very bad time, and her emotions ran roughshod over everything.

When the dust finally settled she said, sadly, "I feel as if three months of my life have been taken away, just when I was beginning to get it back."

It's not lost," I reassured her. "You've worked too hard for it to be lost. It's just been sidelined for a while."

She nodded, but I could see the anguish in her eyes.

PERTINENT POINTS FROM CHAPTER SEVEN

Coping skills also include **getting things in order** and establishing **priorities.**

The way we use **language** affects our emotional responses, and therefore our physiological responses, to a very great degree.

Self-talk is constant and, too often, extremely negative.

It is possible to deliberately **change one's language,** and this promotes healing.

Cognitive changes are vital to understanding chronic pain. They include **behavior modification.**

Feeling **out of control** adds to the desperation of the chronic pain patient.

Reclaiming control includes assertiveness, negotiation, openness, decision making, participation, and reassessment. It also includes dealing with the "what-if" tendency, softening sabotage, managing the comfort, and once again becoming "**the lead dancer.**"

Emotions play a huge role and require appreciation of their **real message.**

Anger is one of the most difficult, and most important emotions to acknowledge.

The roots of anger are **frustration, fear, intrusion** and **injustice.**

WORKSHEET FOR CHAPTER SEVEN

1. Have you used any of the coping skills discussed in this chapter?

2. If so, which ones have worked best for you?

3. Have you used other coping skills which have not been discussed?

4. What are they?

5. How have they worked for you?

6. Jot down some relevant facts about control issues in your particular situation—areas where you may feel you are out of control, or are being controlled:

7. What negative factors can you identify in your situation?

8. How can you start changing any negative factors?

9. Which of your ego states exert the most control?

10. How do they do this?

11. What emotional factors most affect you?

12. How?

13. What negative emotions can you identify?

14. What can you do to start changing negative emotions?

15. How can you use your own self-talk to enhance positive emotions?

16. Begin to explore the role(s) of anger in your own situation:

17. With which root of anger is each part most identified? (frustration, fear, intrusion, or injustice.)

18. With which outside dancers do these angry parts interact?

19. Determine which of these interactions needs to be changed.

20. How are you going to do that?

CHAPTER EIGHT

HARMONY AND HEALING AT LAST!

A New Dance

Harmony: when you look up the word in the dictionary, you find it defined in lovely terms of melodious sound, agreement, concord, and adding notes to form chords. To harmonize, the verb form, is defined as "to bring into harmony; add notes to (melody); to form chords."

It is an **active** process. Harmony doesn't just happen, it must be arranged—by adding and combining notes, by forming chords, by agreement.

So when one has been reduced to an undulating blob of agony because of relentless pain, how could one speak in terms of "achieving harmony"?

Throughout this book, we've talked about 'inside dancers,' or ego states, and 'outside dancers.' The inside *and* outside aspect of achieving harmony are central to the theme. One cannot create a melodious sound if one is all jangling inside, nor in discord with the world outside.

What might one do, in terms of applying some of the approaches we've talked about, to promote more harmony?

I think the metaphor of the choreography gives us a 'window of opportunity' to begin to appreciate the *discord*, and therefore discover where one could begin to alter the scene, ever so slightly to begin with, toward *concord*. Discordant music creates an entirely different dance effect than harmonious music does. With a little internal exploration, you can discover which parts of you relate most quickly and easily to such possibilities.

By contrast, which self-parts/ego states are the hold-outs? It is the hold-outs which we wish to draw gently into the harmony (adding more notes!). Why are some parts holding out? What is the need that is being fulfilled by maintaining tension and discord? Until you investigate the reasons why, things are bound to remain in the minor chords. (Mind you, this may be a great improvement over the total discord with which you had started.)

It would be nice to think that we could get somewhere by changing the *outside* dancers, but of course, that's not possible. All we can do is *change our relationship to them.* That's why the director(s) may very well be some person or persons on the outside, but the choreographer is so often within us. It is the choreographer who truly defines the dance.

> Paul had begun at the pain clinic at the insistence of his doctor. He only went because he couldn't bear the thought of having to find yet another physician—he had already broken off acrimoniously with two others. But they were all so *pompous* and *arrogant!*
>
> His emotional baggage was wrapped in rage. He knew it, but he had no idea what to do about it.
>
> Paul had been a police officer who had been shot in the line of duty. The nerves in his left thigh were badly damaged. He was in the rehab hospital for months—almost a year, actually—and even now his walking wasn't as good as it should be, especially when he was tired.
>
> The weakness bothered him, but it was nothing compared to the pain. The pain was with him all the time, waking and sleeping (not that he slept very much). He had been given honorable retirement from the police force when it became obvious that he was never going to be able to perform his duties again. They *had* offered him a desk job. He turned it down flat.
>
> It is not too hard to see where the roots of Paul's anger

lay. He even knew it himself, intellectually. But knowing it with his rational mind didn't even make a dent in his fierce emotional response.

Part of the protocol at the pain clinic was to have regular sessions with one of the psychologists. He was assigned to a woman. A woman! As if she could possibly have the dimmest glimmer of what he had gone through—was going through! But protocol was protocol. If there was anything he had learned in all his years with the police, it was how to follow orders. So he went, dutifully, and sat with closed ears and guarded mind.

"Paul," she finally said to him one day, "**I am not your enemy!** Your enemy is within you. Not me, not even the man who shot you. Something within *you*. Until we find out what that is, you will constantly undermine all that we hope to achieve here. Is that what you want?"

He was caught completely off-balance. "N-no, of—of course not," he stammered. (What is wrong with me? he thought. I can't even talk straight.)

"Good. That's what I believe, too. So let's make a contract. You let me in, just a little bit, to that place of anger and pain. You can choose how much, but it has to be *some*. Will you agree?"

Slowly, he nodded.

"Agreed, then. And, whatever that small inroad is, we will work with it until we understand it and can let the gate open a bit wider. Are we agreed again?"

He nodded.

"Right. Our time is up for today, but there is some homework for you. You have to talk to yourself and find out how much it will be okay to disclose to me—about your feelings, your fear, your rage. Because that's where your pain is. And it will never even begin to go away until the fear and the rage are accepted for what they are, and dealt with. So you have a little inside chat, and when you come next time, you can tell me—whatever you are ready to tell me. Okay?"

"Okay." Feeling slightly stunned, he left her office.

This unfinished vignette epitomizes much of what we have been considering throughout this book. It encapsulates transference issues, seething emotions, rage of the 'injustice' caliber, contracts, making small changes, assertive confrontation (in this case from the psychologist, but Paul will get into the act in time), internal dialogue between some of Paul's ego states, outside dancers, and the initial phase of adding notes to the chords, to name just a few aspects. It's too soon to talk about harmony—that's a long way down the road for Paul. But the discordant choreography *has* begun to change.

We are adding notes to the melody and starting to create harmonious chords when we explore some new techniques, be they cognitive, behavioral, or those which are directed to the subconscious. Every time we do, something changes. (It is impossible to change something—anything—within a system and not have everything else shuffle around, too.) As the music changes, so does The Dance.

When situations go on and on, seemingly forever, it is hard to recognize such changes. It takes concerted effort, directed effort, to continuously reassess a situation in order to appreciate these tiny moves. This does not mean frantically looking for some evidence of change every day, but rather, sitting down for some quiet time, for instance, every couple of weeks or so and allowing the recognition of some new movement in The Dance to become clearer.

Other people in our lives often perceive these changes earlier than we do. Close family, one's mate/spouse/partner, the family doctor, friends whom you trust, sometimes colleagues at work— theirs are the more objective eyes which may have seen something that we, with our totally subjective view, haven't.

Sometimes, when there is still a fair amount of internal sabotage at work, we may deny such observations, believing self-righteously that others are only seeing the façade. Of course, that may be true, and many people have an amazing outer presentation that in no way reflects their inner torture; but don't discount those observations which are made without the burden of the suffering. Just listen, accept that that is what someone has noticed, and file it away until you are ready to consider it from the inside.

Here are some examples:

- Edith's doctor notices that her calls to him have not been quite as frequent for the past few weeks. (Only a couple of times a week instead of almost every day.) Edith believes that she has never called him that often.

- Bob notices that his wife, Sue, doesn't need to call him at work so often to ask him to pick up her prescription at the drug store. (She seems to be able to make the pills last until the weekend.) Sue believes that Bob is exaggerating again—maybe she asked him to pick it up once or twice.

- Henry's coworker notices that Henry seems to be getting through the day better. (It used to be that, by five o'clock, the lines of pain were etched into Henry's face.) Henry believes that he has never allowed his pain to show on his face—that would be tantamount to asking for pity.

- David's mother, with whom he has lived since his divorce, notices that he doesn't seem to prowl the house late at night so much. (She's sure that he used to spend most of the night going over and over the break-up of his marriage, which he attributed directly to his accident.) David believes that he has dealt well with the divorce right from the beginning—after all, you couldn't expect someone to stay with a cripple.

In time, Edith, Sue, Henry and David will be ready to at least entertain the possibility that their attitudes have modified somewhat, perhaps allowing some new rhythms in the music of The Dance. Right now, it's too soon. That's okay, but it's important that they be given the feedback so that they can file it away safely within the subconscious for a while yet. Edith's doctor, Bob, Henry's co-worker, and David's mother can realize that it is just too risky for their patient/wife/colleague/son to begin to believe that things might be getting a little easier. What if it's just a fleeting moment of release, which will be taken away from them again if they start to count on it?

For people who have been imprisoned by the choreography of pain, it's often safer to let it happen gradually; and it *will* happen gradually, but it is still important for the sufferers to allow a little elasticity in their responses—just take that time, every so often, to look back and think about what *may* be different. In time you can begin to realize how far you've come.

HOW WILL I KNOW WHEN THINGS ARE DIFFERENT?

Look back, with honest appraisal, to six months before, and compare.

Listen when someone tells you that they've noticed something.

Keep a journal so that you can compare today with last month.

Pay attention to your *feelings* when it seems that today wasn't such a bad day.

Realize that you're sleeping better.

Monitor any medication that you may be taking; discuss it with your doctor if you think you may not need so much.

Appreciate it if your appetite has improved.

Recognize that you can rely on your energy level to be higher during certain times each day.

These are all markers which can indicate that The Dance is changing, even just a little bit. But the best way to discern such modifications in your own choreography is to **check things out with your inside dancers, *often!*** Ask *them* what has changed. Get the dialogues going, and make sure those dialogues are vigorous and positive.

Remember Marie, way back in Chapter Four? Let's see what might have changed for her.

Perhaps she has begun to reject being identified as "the patient" and has re-identified herself as a woman who happens to have pain; it interferes with her life, but she *has* a life.

Maybe she has had a good talk with herself and realized that there are times when someone does need help from other people and that those others do not perceive it in the same negative "asking for favors" way that she does.

It's possible that the "positive-angry" self has assumed a stronger role in the dance and has learned to be assertive with disability evaluators, lawyers, doctors, etc. She recognizes facts, but also makes sure that *her* needs are recognized.

She might now allow that having been a wonderful, competent teacher will always be part of her and that there may be, in the future, a further opportunity for this competent part of her to be involved in teaching in some way.

Perhaps she has had some heart-to-hearts with Tim, and has begun to assuage her unrealistic guilt.

These are just some of the ways in which her ego states could be modifying their roles, making use of their particular talents.

Presuming that some of this is happening—and we can presume that possibility, because Marie is an intelligent woman who does want to do those things—then we can think of what effect those things will have on the outside dancers.

There's no question, for instance, that Tim would appreciate being allowed back into the situation in some more helpful way; or that Marie's doctors would respond positively to her reasonable assertiveness. Although she cannot *make* outside dancers change, they *will* change in response to her changes—again, once something moves in a system, everything else must move too.

On the other hand, is it possible that none of these hopeful things have happened and that she's sinking further into the mire? Sure, it's possible. Not only that, it is almost inevitable *until and unless she makes a committed effort to prevent it.*

That committed effort is the bottom line for everyone carrying the yoke of chronic pain. It means **allowing the possibility of positive change,** even when you cannot see how or where it could begin to happen. Here is where a good solid streak of stubbornness really helps.

Believe in yourself. You are the best resource you could possibly have.

Samantha came in looking very pleased with herself, despite the fact that she obviously had a headache.

She had been applying her new awarenesses in practical ways, and the results were surprising both to her and to Dave.

"Dave told me that I'm going to have to be more careful with my pills," she said.

Was that an alarm bell? "What do you mean?" I asked.

She grinned at me. "It's because he's finding pills all over the house, in the car—it worries him. He thinks I'm being very careless."

I waited. There was obviously something I was missing here.

"You see," she explained, "I always used to make sure that I had some pills handy, wherever I might be. I would take a few and put them in a little package and stash them. Even if I went into a different room, I might take some pills with me. But now, I'm finding them still there!"

Apparently she had also been surprised to find that, when the usual time came to renew one of her prescriptions, she still had a significant number left. And that happened the next time she went to renew them, too. A major change!

"And," she confided, "a few times I've put a couple of pills in my pocket, planning to take them in a few minutes; and after a while, I'll be feeling pleased that the pills have worked and the pain has gone away—and then I'd find the pills still in my pocket! I hadn't even taken them!"

No wonder she was so pleased with herself.

Dancing to harmony is totally different from dancing to jarring, abstract, atonal, discordant sound.

This does not mean that there will no longer be a dance going on that is connected to those old soul-shaking blasts: obviously, there *is*, and a dreadful dance it may be, in the sense of how one responds to such images. Some modern dance is like that. It is meant to jolt us from our complacency, force us to look at something we might prefer not to see. In fulfilling that purpose, it can be highly effective.

Translate that into the situation of chronic pain—perhaps your own situation.

Imagine how the demands of that harsh discord sap your energy, invade your life. There seems to be no escape.

We've been considering, throughout this book, a variety of possibilities for identifying that escape route. They all lie within us, so to explore them we have to explore within. Much as we all long for magic, there is none. There is only hard work, and dedication, and honesty, and a glimmer of light at the end of the tunnel.

Samantha's day-to-day world was slowing but surely changing.

She was, indeed, "managing the comfort instead of the pain." She had enjoyed her gardening during the summer and had lots of preserves to show for it. And she was happily into her quilting, finishing some projects that had been around for months (or years). She was generating new quilting patterns, leading workshops, and having a great time.

"I have *chunks* of time, now," she told me. "It's something new—I haven't had chunks of time, pain-free time, for years and years and years. And another thing—the pattern is really changing; the mornings are usually just fine, no pain at all. If I'm going to get a headache, it will often not come on until well into the afternoon. It's great, because then I can just go to bed after supper and sleep it off and I'm fine in the morning."

Samantha has taken back control of her life. She is comfortable with the fact that it is too soon to even think about going back to work. She and Dave have reappraised their lives and made some changes in their priorities. She has talked to her mother about her concerns. Her inside and outside dancers have embarked on new dance routines which encourage them to interact in different ways from the old responses.

She knows that there is still a lot of work to do. But in fact, she has evolved—and she continues to evolve—a whole new choreography.

And that's what it's all about.

PERTINENT POINTS FROM CHAPTER EIGHT

Changing the choreography involves moving from discord to **harmony** within.

Such change can never come from outside: **It can only come from within.**

There are usually internal "hold-outs" which can sabotage change.

Achieving more harmony requires **positive internal dialogue.**

CHANGE IS POSSIBLE!

WORKSHEET FOR CHAPTER EIGHT

1. Which ego states could be your internal "hold-outs"?

2. Why might they be holding out? What could be the need?

3. How can you begin to persuade them to change?

4. Evaluate your internal dialogues. Who are the main participants?

5. How can you ensure that your self-talk stays positive?

CHAPTER NINE

RESEARCH AND LITERATURE REVIEW AND COMMENTARIES

Because this book is directed toward both those who suffer chronic pain and those who wish to help such sufferers, it seemed to me to be important to include some examples of recent research and literature, with a brief commentary about them.

Some readers who are not medically or psychologically inclined may find the excerpts heavy sledding. (Some of us who *are* medically or psychologically inclined find some of them heavy sledding, too!) But I hope that there will be some information in this chapter of interest to every reader.

It is by no means a comprehensive review: it's meant to whet your appetite, to give you some inkling about the state of the art in chronic pain concepts and treatment.

The excerpts are arranged alphabetically by author. A short bibliography of other books you may find interesting appears at the end.

Barton, P. M. (1995) Chronic pain management for the family practitioner. *The Canadian Journal of CME,* **August: pp. 73–83.**

Dr. Barton, a clinical associate professor in the division of physical medicine and rehabilitation at the University of Calgary, presents a definitive outline of the integrated approach, especially the team approach, in a chronic pain rehabilitation program. She points out that the earlier treatment is initiated, the more favorable the result is likely to be. This paper focuses more on the family physician and his or her frustration at being able to offer such limited possibilities of "cure" to chronic pain patients, with consequent countertransference issues in dealing with desperate sufferers. She offers practical, down-to-earth advice on management including examples of management plans and an information sheet for patients.

COMMENTARY

The aspect of the physician's emotional response to the patient's obvious desperation and suffering is seldom referred to in the literature in such a specific way. This aspect of the interaction—an important scene in the choreography—needs to be more fully explored for the benefit of doctor AND patient.

Catchlove, R. F. H. (1991) A guide to diagnosis and management of chronic pain. *The Canadian Journal of CME*, Nov–Dec: pp. 33–41.

Breaking down chronic pain into its component modalities will allow rational choices as to which of the treatment approaches will be the most appropriate and useful. The author points out, "Chronic pain patients typically describe interference with their life activities of more than 50%; they miss or are unable to work; sports and other activities are abandoned or greatly reduced; social interactions are diminished; family relationships and structures are severely distorted; and depression is frequent."

Most chronic pain patients have been very active and hardworking before the onset of the pain; malingering or lying is not congruent with their usual lifestyle and therefore very unlikely.

Dr. Catchlove states that the neuroanatomic pathways which transmit acute pain are the same as those which perceive and transmit chronic pain. This is a complicated system, polyneuronal and polysynaptic, with the presence of both long and short feedback loops, the release of multiple neurotransmitters, intraspinal inter-segmental activity, and lateral input. "An appreciation of the function of feedback loops does provide a conceptual framework for the understanding of chronic pain of a mixed physical and psychological origin."

He describes the integral involvement of the limbic system, which is crucial to the understanding of the altered perception of pain experienced by chronic pain patients. He believes that the incidence of alexithymia (lack of words to express emotions) is much higher in chronic pain sufferers than in the general population and extends this to the concept that these patients express their emotions through pain. "Viewed from this perspective, chronic pain patients may be considered as suffering a communication disorder."

The article goes on to elaborate a comprehensive approach through a multimodal treatment program which includes physiotherapy, nerve blocks, medication, neuro-ablative procedures, psychotherapy, other therapies such as art, occupational, and work retraining and, finally, maintenance.

COMMENTARY

Two important points from this excellent article are:

That the neuroanatomic pathways which transmit acute pain are the same as those which perceive and transmit chronic pain;

That the limbic system is integrally involved in these neuroanatomic pathways.

These points are central to the hypothesis of the choreography of chronic pain which is the metaphor in this book. If the neuroanatomic pathways are the same, then it must be that the *perception* is different; and since the limbic system is so integrally involved, it is congruent to extend this fact to the necessary involvement of the emotional and psychological factors which attend chronic pain *which are different from those which attend acute pain*, as being key factors in this difference in perception.

Crasilneck, H. B. (1995) The use of the Crasilneck Bombardment Technique in problems of intractable pain. *American Journal of Clinical Hypnosis, 37, 4,* pp. 255–266.

Crasilneck describes several patients who had come to him for chronic pain problems, who had not responded to conventional therapies, and who also had not responded to the usual hypnotic interventions.

He therefore devised a "Bombardment Technique," comprised of relaxation, displacement, age regression, glove anaesthesia, hypnoanaesthesia and self-hypnosis. The patient is "bombarded" with these techniques in hour-long sessions, each segment lasting seven to ten minutes. The treatment program is very time-consuming and must be preplanned, with a patient committed to follow it through.

Successful outcomes, which lasted over time, are described in patients who were previously refractory to all therapeutic approaches.

COMMENTARY

Dr. Crasilneck is one of the most venerable members of the international clinical hypnosis community, highly regarded for the breadth of his clinical experience and his understanding of hypnotic phenomena. It seems to me that in this paper he is attesting to the fact that chronic pain syndromes require special approaches and combinations of techniques that in other less arduous conditions would more likely be effective when used separately.

Crawford, H. J. (1995) Brain dynamic shifts during hypnotic analgesia: Why can't we all eliminate pain? Paper presented at the 37th Annual Meeting of the American Society of Clinical Hypnosis, San Diego.

In her splendid plenary presentation, Dr. Crawford described the frontolimbic attentional system for both attending to and ignoring stimuli in one's environment (internal and external environments). She postulated that perhaps highly hypnotizable individuals may have a more efficient system for frontal lobe activities and—as an extension of that possibility—that chronic pain patients, who seem to be supersensitive to pain stimuli, might be more highly hypnotizable than the general population.

As the frontal lobe mediates motivational-affective and sensory-discrimination information, and its activities could be considered to include those of executive controller, regulating sequential action and behavior, maintaining sustained focused attention, controlling inhibitory processes and allowing disattention, the question arises: is this *capacity* or *process*? Can we develop neurobiofeedback?

COMMENTARY

The concept that chronic pain patients may be more sensitive to pain stimuli than the general population, and that they also may be more hypnotizable, is intriguing. It offers a theory which might account for the enigma of why some people develop chronic pain syndromes and others do not.

Should this idea be further explored, it might also offer opportunities for earlier interventions, so important in preventing the slide into chronic pain—for instance, using hypnotic interventions to foster ignoring, rather than attending to, the stimuli.

Crawford, H. J. (1995) Use of hypnotic techniques in the control of pain: Neuropsychophysiological foundations and evidence. Paper presented at the Technology and Assessment Conference on Integration of Behavioral and Relaxation Approaches into the Treatment of Chronic Pain and Insomnia, National Institute of Health, Natcher Conference Center, October 16–18.

This paper describes, with reference to research similar to that cited above, ways in which people can use imagery, distraction, and relaxation techniques in order to reduce or even eliminate "*perception* of distress and sensory pain." Dr. Crawford points out that, once these techniques are learned, they can be adapted to other, non-hypnotic, contexts.

Referring to Melzak's work, she comments that we still do not fully understand how hypnosis can so dramatically and quickly reduce "what appear to be strongly developed neurosignatures of pain."

In her conclusion, Dr. Crawford asserts that "Hypnosis and other psychological interventions need to be introduced *early* as adjuncts in medical treatments for pain—before the development of strong pain memories and before surgery and long regimens of drug treatment, not after."

COMMENTARY

Dr. Crawford's concluding comments are particularly important for our work with chronic pain. So often, the patient is already enveloped in the chronic syndrome before such non-surgical, non-pharmaceutical approaches are even introduced.

In the early chapters of this book I commented on how important it was to stop *persistent pain* from spiraling down the helpless/hopeless slope into chronic pain. This excellent paper confirms that importance.

Finer, B. (1995) Whiplash injury and hypnotherapy. *Hypnos,* *XXII,* *1:* pp. 32–38.

This paper refers to the "chronic sickness cultures," of which chronic pain (in these cases, following whiplash) is a prime example. Dr. Finer points out that in such situations, the sickness (the pain), the rehabilitation, and the reality of the chronic patient differ fundamentally from those of healthy people, and that this very fact accounts for much of the feelings of confusion and alienation which is experienced by chronic pain patients. He refers to becoming a chronic pain patient as a "culture shock of considerable magnitude." With miserable paradox, the "healthy person's culture" (society, and the medical community) controls the "pain person's culture."

He also discusses the formation of "subpersonalities" which react and respond amongst themselves and with other people.

In discussing hypnotherapy, Finer refers to the importance of establishing a "common language of communication" in order to better understand the imagery of the patient's personal inner world, secure trust, and create appropriate metaphor. He suggests describing the feelings of helplessness as destructive and negative and replacing them with positive suggestions of successful rehabilitation.

COMMENTARY

The identification of chronic pain experience in *cultural* terms is a new approach, and one that makes a great deal of sense. Finding oneself to be suddenly "hopeless and helpless," in the chronic pain vortex, can indeed be thought of as a culture shock of considerable magnitude. Such a situation can certainly be described as a type of posttraumatic stress disorder.

Dr. Finer and I have frequently discussed the similarities of our concepts of chronic pain phenomena, (e.g., my "inside and outside dancers" and his "subpersonalities.") He also adapts a "company board" metaphor which facilitates the inner participants in their communication with each other.

Earlier in the book I referred to Dr. Finer's multidisciplinary pain clinic in Sweden. Within the clinic he puts all these concepts into active practice.

Flor, H., Birbaumer, N., Schugens, M. M., and Lutzenberger, W. (1992) Symptom-specific psychophysiological responses in chronic pain patients. *Psychophysiology, 29,* 4: pp. 452–460.

The authors assessed 20 chronic back pain patients, 20 temporomandibular pain and dysfunction patients, and 20 healthy controls. The hypothesis was that stressful environmental stimuli may provoke specific physiological responses; in this study, the investigated response was EMG reactivity and hyperreactivity in chronic pain patients.

The authors explain their specificity approach based on a previously proposed model, of which a central component is that chronic musculoskeletal pain syndromes develop from and also can be exacerbated by the interaction of potentially stressful events, inadequate coping skills/abilities, and a predisposing organic or psychological condition, or diathesis. If such stimuli is intense and/or recurrent, in the absence of adequate coping skills, such a patient may develop a "response stereotypy" in a vulnerable physiological system.

Such vulnerability could be due to several factors: over-use of certain muscle groups (e.g., neck and shoulders in typists), a structural problem such as spondylolisthesis,* or an acute injury; it could, the authors propose, also be due to "observational learning." The authors state: "This individual response stereotypy may manifest itself as a local muscular hyperreaction that may become prolonged the more dysregulated the individual's physiological system becomes. Homeostatic failure may ensue if the overreaction of the system occurs on a regular basis."

Flor *et al* found that chronic back pain patients responded with marked EMG increases in the erector spinae musculature, and also a prolonged return to baseline, when discussing stressful life events or pain episodes, but not when doing something emotionally neutral such as reciting the alphabet. These increases were not seen in the control group.

The authors found that, for patients with TMJ pain and for patients with chronic back pain, reactivity in response to discussing emotionally stressful situations was increased *at the site of the pain* but not at other, more distal sites. Although the changes in microvolts were small, the authors point out that these changes were in response to an *imagined* stressor, and they hypothesize that actual stressors outside the laboratory may evoke a much greater response.

They also found an unexpected result: there were significant negative correlations between heart rate reactivity and a helpless attitude toward pain, in contrast to positive heart rate reactivity and an active coping attitude. They suggest further research into this observation.

The authors conclude: ". . . these results provide evidence for a localized overresponding of the pain-related muscles to personally relevant stressful stimulation—imagined or real. These results do not confirm a concept of tonic generalized tension and arousal

---

*Spondylolisthesis is a condition in which an upper vertebra slides forward over a lower one, instead of sitting on it squarely and securely.

in chronic pain patients. Therefore, assessments of chronic pain patients should include the measurement of site- and symptom-specific psychophysiological response to stress."

COMMENTARY

This excellent article attends to a different aspect of the chronic pain patient's dilemma. Not only does the patient have a chronic pain syndrome, but the EMG hyperresponse (which manifests itself as increased pain) is worsened *at the site of the pain* by that person's response to stressful situations. This, in turn, is worsened if the patient has poor coping skills. Two of the authors further their observations in the following article.

Flor, H. and Birbaumer, N. (1994) Acquisition of chronic pain: Psychophysiological mechanisms. *APS Journal, 3, (2):* **pp. 119–127.**

The premise of the authors is that psychophysiological mechanisms play an important role in both the development and maintenance of chronic pain syndromes. They suggest that those patients who are most at risk to develop chronic pain states have either already experienced a pain-related conditioning, and/or they have a predisposition to respond to painful stimulation with what they call "enhanced conditionability."

They found in earlier studies that some chronic pain patients show deficits in the perception of changes in muscle tension, and that that may contribute to a delayed return to baseline of muscle tension. They assert that such changes must be central in origin because they are present in muscles unrelated to the pain site. Furthermore, lower pain thresholds and lower pain tolerance have been observed in chronic pain patients (e.g., chronic back pain) but not in patients with episodic pain (e.g., recurrent headaches).

The authors believe that these alterations in the processing of both external and internal pain-related stimulation are related to cortical pain memories (similar to Melzak's "neurosignature").

Furthermore, they state that "Operant and respondent learning processes form explicit [and] also many implicit memories that the person is not aware of but which have profound influences

on perception and motor action. . . . These memories also influence pain perception and pain behaviour."

To support these hypotheses, they used nonlinear EEG analy-
sis, and found that in chronic pain patients, the memory of a pain
event elicited a significantly higher dimensional complexity of the
EEG than it did in healthy controls. They pointed out that such
responses were specific to *personally relevant pain and stress
episodes*: similar responses were not elicited from suggested sce-
narios. Therefore the "enhanced responses are not simply non-
specific reflex responses to stress but may have been conditioned
to pain-relevant stimuli."

COMMENTARY

If ever a work supported the theory of "body memories," this
work does. It is particularly important that the premise is supported by the scientific data. The concept of chronic pain patients
being conditioned in their response to painful stimuli makes it
even more important that early interventions based on psychophysiological awareness be employed, as soon as there is the
faintest suggestion of persistent—leading to chronic—pain behavior.

**Gerecz-Simon, E. M., Kean, W. F., and Buchanan, W. W.
(1991) New criteria for the classification of fibromyalgia.
Canadian Journal of Diagnosis, February: pp. 80–96.**

This paper identifies fibromyalgia as occurring in 10% to 15%
of the population, and 10 times more often in women than in
men. The diagnostic parameters are specific and include 18 trigger points, and a necessity for four-quadrant plus axial pain. They
describe other frequent co-morbidity characteristics such as sleep
disturbance, fatigue, paraesthesiae, headache, and dysmenor-
rhoea. They specifically refer to alpha non-REM sleep anomaly,
characterized on EEG. Laboratory findings include decreased serotonin levels, low natural killer cell activity, increased Substance P
in the CSF and elevated serum interleukin-2 activity.

They outline a comprehensive but realistic differential diagnosis, and a management program which focuses on lifestyle and pain relief techniques such as biofeedback, relaxation techniques, and transcutaneous electric nerve stimulation.

COMMENTARY

This excellent paper addresses the fear of all patients that their doctors will think their pain is 'all in her head,' and therefore makes very specific and comprehensive commentary on those diagnostic criteria which ARE specific and measurable. It is infinitely helpful for patients to be able to hear and read about such specific signs and symptoms, thus validating their experience. Tension over whether one's medical advisor believes or disbelieves one's pain experience can add immeasurably to the pain. Gerecz-Simon and her colleagues do much to allay that fear.

Hall, H., McIntosh, G., and Melles, T. (1995) Recognition and management of the chronic pain syndrome. *The Canadian Journal of CME,* March: pp. 39–48.

Dr. Hamilton Hall is known as "The Back Doctor." He has written extensively on back pain and its management. In this article, he and his colleagues from The Canadian Back Institute describe chronic pain syndrome as ". . . a behavioural disorder. It is a pattern of abnormal behaviour in which pain becomes the patient's primary focus and the principal determinant of all activity."

The authors point out that one of the most damaging misperceptions regarding chronic pain syndrome is the idea that the pain is not real. They reassert that all pain is real, and that patients with pain perception problems (an increased awareness of sensory input) are not malingering, and that their reaction to pain is not under voluntary control. They also state that ". . . there are no consistently valid indicators of a patient's vulnerability. It is best to assume that anyone, given the necessary circumstances, can succumb to this behavioural abnormality."

They comment on the many possible exacerbating factors, such as sleep disturbances (*very* important—they believe that if sleep disturbance is not part of the history, the diagnosis is in doubt), mechanical pain, pain arising from uncomplicated soft tissue lesions, excessive medical involvement, sexual dysfunction, and family disruption, "circumstantial pain syndrome," and pertinent aspects of the physical examination, which are described in detail.

Management is focused on *shifting the patient's attention to the pain, to a more productive area*, thus breaking the patient's learned behavioral response; and in scrupulously attending to the parameters of sleep, mechanical factors, sexual dysfunction, disruption of family relationships, medication (almost always useless), and the detrimental effect of pain on all aspects of the patient's life.

COMMENTARY

Hall, McIntosh and Melles define chronic pain as a *behavioral* disorder, rather than as Catchlove's definition of a *communication* disorder. The concept, nevertheless, is very much the same. Both fit equally well into the metaphor of choreography. Both advise strongly that altering learned behavior patterns and responses are crucial if one is going to achieve relief from any chronic pain syndrome. Both assert strongly that chronic pain, as any other pain, is real, and wipe away the stigma that somehow the chronic pain patient is more vulnerable (i.e., somehow deficient to such a situation—or, to put it even more boldly, that the patient is to blame for his or her pain).

Hart, M. (1993) Silken steel. *Body and soul,* Spring: pp. 16–22.

This is a vivid account of the injuries which were sustained by Silken Laumann, the Olympic gold medalist, while she was training for the Barcelona Olympics in 1992.

Laumann was, at that time, the world's top woman scull racer. She and many other competitors were warming up for an international racing event in Germany. One of the other sculls crashed into her—she does not hold any blame towards them—slicing the muscles away from the bone in her lower right leg.

She received excellent immediate care in Germany and was flown home to Victoria, British Columbia, four days later.

Everybody thought that her competition in the Olympics, just a short 10 weeks away, was impossible. Instead, she and her coaches and medical team worked through an agonizing, incredible regime of rehabilitation. The intense motivation of all concerned—to completely ignore pain, to focus totally on strengthening the lacerated muscles—paid off. Two months later, she won the bronze medal at the Barcelona Olympics.

COMMENTARY

Ms. Laumann's astonishing achievement testifies to the depths of inner strength upon which a person can draw, in working *through* decimating pain when the goal is sufficiently central to one's sense of self and self-fulfillment. It is when this sense of self is eroded by persistent pain that the specter of a chronic pain syndrome arises.

Katz, J. (1992) Psychophysical correlates of phantom limb experience. *Journal of Neurology, Neurosurgery and Psychiatry, 55,* 9: pp. 811–821.

Katz, J. (1993) Psychophysiological contributions to phantom limbs. *Canadian Journal of Psychiatry, 37,* 5: pp. 282–298.

These two papers describe Dr. Katz' work in establishing that true phantom limb pain (as differentiated from other types of discomfort) only exists when there has been significant pain *prior* to the amputation, and the phantom pain experienced is similar in intensity and location to that earlier pain.

COMMENTARY

In my book *Creative Scripts for Hypnotherapy,* I referred to the contributions of this top researcher in the field of phantom limb pain. In the first paper, he described earlier work with Melzack which specifically discussed a type of phantom pain which is experienced in the survivor as the same or very similar pain, in location and quality, to that which had been experienced before the amputation. I noted that "According to Dr. Katz, the data offer strong further indication that pain which is experienced prior to amputation may persist in the form of somatosensory memory in the phantom limb. He discusses input from the sympathetic nervous system, psychological and emotional factors, and what he describes as somatosensory reorganization. These studies have important implications for anyone working with pain, especially chronic pain syndromes, and with abuse and trauma survivors."

Katz' work was predicated on earlier work by Melzack, who had brought out an updated hypothesis, described below.

Kropotov, J. D., Crawford, H. J., and Polyakov, Y. I. (1996) Somatosensory event-related potential changes to painful stimuli during hypnotic analgesia: Anterior cingulate cortex and anterior temporal cortex intracranial recordings in obsessive-compulsives. (In press, *International Journal of Psychophysiology*.)

The authors believe that this study is the first to demonstrate the involvement of the anterior cingulate cortex and the anterior temporal cortex in the control of pain through hypnoanalgesia. They referred to the hypothesis that people who are highly hypnotizable may have a stronger attention filter to distracting stimuli which are associated with the fronto-attentional directional system, and that this capability permits them to inhibit painful stimuli more effectively than people who have lower hypnotizability.

They point out that the anterior cingulate cortex, prefrontal cortex, thalamus, and amygdala, interconnected, are implicated in attentional processes as well as in numerous other activities, including pain and emotion. They quote one study in which "Ablations to the rostral cingulum bundle [led] to patients reporting sensory pain perception with lack of discomfort or distress."

Their research followed changes in the somatosensory event-related potentials (SERPs), anticipating that there would be changes recorded from anterior regions of the brain when hypnotic analgesia was introduced. This expectation was fulfilled. Further support for their hypothesis was provided by their work on regional cerebral blood flow while attending and disattending to stimuli (see Crawford (1995) citation, pp. 150–151).

COMMENTARY

This study is an example of the elegant and sophisticated research which is being done in this field. It is exceedingly detailed, and the scientific language is certainly not in everyone's repertoire, but it is a supremely important work.

When Dr. Crawford referred to this work in her plenary talk, she pointed out that the more highly hypnotizable person may have more active control over inhibitory processes, and also possibly a more effective fronto-limbic attentional system.

This is different from the situation where one changes his or her *response* to the pain, e.g., through shifting emphasis away from the pain—in other words, through changing the choreography.

The authors' conclusion, that "multiple brain stems contribute to pain and to the development of hypnotic analgesia," is particularly important (from our perspective here) when they also relate those systems to emotion.

Large, R. G. (1994) Hypnosis for chronic pain: A critical review. *Hypnos, XXI,* **4: pp. 234–237.**

Although countless papers have been written and presented about the relief of chronic pain through hypnosis, most of these are anecdotal and very few evaluate this modality in any systematic way; even fewer describe some form of experimental control.

This paper offers a review of that literature which does attend to these parameters. The author's conclusion, after evaluating twelve papers, is that hypnosis is an effective therapy in the management of chronic pain but may not be any more effective than autogenic training or relaxation techniques. A strong plea is made for more detailed studies which adhere to scientific principles.

COMMENTARY

Dr. Large, in Auckland, New Zealand, is known for his work on chronic pain. Although he supports and teaches the use of hypnotic interventions for the relief of chronic pain syndromes, he deplores the fact that publication in the field of clinical hypnosis is frequently anecdotal; he feels that this weakens the status of this discipline. Therefore, while using these techniques himself, he maintains very rigorous standards both in his own papers and in those which he recommends, in order to maintain maximum credibility.

He will no doubt be extremely interested in some of the literature I have reviewed in this book, which certainly does attend to scientific controlled studies involving hypnoanalgesia for the relief of pain and, in particular, chronic pain.

Machan, L. (1995) Work reported in *The Vancouver Sun*, April 13, by Health Editor, Rebecca Wigod.

Dr. Lindsay Machan has been working with women with pelvic pain syndrome, a type of chronic pain condition which intensifies over time and which some doctors deny exists. He has developed a treatment for this condition when it is due to pelvic varicose veins, especially those near the ovaries. Women with this condition find that they are comfortable when they first get up in the morning, but feel increasing pain throughout the day as the upright position allows the veins to become congested with blood. Sexual intercourse is extremely uncomfortable, except in the morning. Dr. Machan treats the condition by inserting, with radiological monitoring, a small catheter into the ovarian vein; if the situation is as he suspected, and there is a backflow of blood causing congestion, he inserts a tiny steel coil to create a clot, preventing the backflow. He stressed that this procedure, "ovarian vein embolization," must not be done until other possible causes for pelvic pain have been investigated thoroughly and ruled out.

COMMENTARY

This is a good example of a situation where women experience chronic pain, in this case in the pelvis, and they are disbelieved or their suffering is minimized until some researcher pays attention. If the situation is NOT corrected, the pain will persist and, of course, get worse as the varicosities enlarge.

Such pain seriously interferes with a woman's functioning, not only with sexual dysfunction (obviously) but also with day-to-day living and working.

A further perspective on chronic pelvic pain syndrome is found in Robinson's work (see Robinson (1994) citation, p. 165).

Melzack, R. (1990) Phantom limbs and the concept of a neuromatrix. *Trends in Neuroscience, 13, 3*: pp. 88–92.

This paper elaborates a new hypothesis for the neural basis of phantom limb phenomena.

Such phenomena are not limited to amputation of a limb or extremity; they have also been described after the surgical removal of the breast or penis. Furthermore, even amputation is not necessary to cause the sensation. Melzack states: "After avulsion of the brachial plexus of the arm, without injury to the arm itself, most patients report a phantom arm (the 'third arm'), which is usually extremely painful. Even nerve destruction is not necessary. About 95% of patients who receive an anaesthesic block of the brachial plexus for surgery of the arm report a vivid phantom, usually at the side or over the chest, which is unrelated to the position of the real arm when the eyes are closed but 'jumps' into it when the patient looks at the arm." Similarly, he points out that a spinal anaesthetic block of the lower body often produces reports of phantom legs in patients, and that a total section of the spinal cord at thoracic levels, e.g., by severe trauma, leads to reports of a phantom body including genitalia and many other body parts in virtually all patients.

The quality of the sensory experiences does not only relate to pain. It also includes touch, pressure, warmth, cold, and even tickle, itchiness, and texture. Full sexual sensations, including orgasm, may be experienced by both men and women paraplegics.

Children who are born without all or part of a limb frequently feel a vivid phantom of the missing part, negating the old belief that phantoms are experienced only if the limb is removed after the age of six or seven years.

In order to form a concept which embodies all of this diverse data, and which accounts for both heredity and environmental factors, Melzack developed the neuromatrix hypothesis. He feels that the explanation must begin in the brain, where ". . . a genetically built-in matrix of neurons for the whole body produces characteristic nerve-impulse patterns for the body and the myriad somatosensory qualities we feel." He goes on to describe how such a matrix, which includes thalamocortical and limbic loops repeatedly converging to permit countless interactions, can (and does) then result in a characteristic "neurosignature."

The paper describes in detail how this concept explains the various phantom phenomena, including those experienced by children born without limbs. He includes a discussion of phantom limb pain and relates it back to the neuromatrix concept.

COMMENTARY

One can see that this hypothesis by Melzack opened the door to a whole new way of looking at phantom experience, and led to Katz' work on phantom pain. It is interesting to extrapolate how one's individual "neurosignature" might be involved in the subsequent experience of "body memories."

Pert, C. (1993) An interview with Bill Moyers in *Healing and the Mind,* originally produced as a PBS television series and subsequently published by Doubleday.

Dr. Candace Pert is perhaps the world's leading researcher on neuropeptides. She is credited with discovering the opiate receptor (and many other peptide receptors) not only within the brain but also throughout the body.

Peptides appear to mediate intercellular communication throughout the body. The theory is that these neuropeptides and their receptors are the *biochemical correlates* of emotions. As they interact, the body responds; and their interactions are constantly changing. "It's a very dynamic, fluid system," says Dr. Pert.

Emotions and physical response are, therefore, inextricably linked. Bill Moyers: "Can our moods and attitudes physically affect our organs and tissues?" Candace Pert: "I believe they can, because moods and attitudes that come from the realm of the mind transform themselves into the physical realm through the emotions."

COMMENTARY

In Dr. Pert's work we have yet another opportunity to consider the physiological responses conjointly with the emotional reactions in body. She makes a very strong case for shifting the old consideration that mind and body, although interacting, are somehow separate, into the concept that emotions are part of the body and physiological response includes emotions.

Such a broadening of the theories of pain helps us to formulate and understand new approaches for the relief of pain. Because of the integral role of emotional response, the focus on relieving the suffering component of chronic pain achieves even more validity.

Robinson, E. (1994) Chronic pelvic pain syndrome. *Psychology in Female Healthcare, 8, 3*: p. 11.

Dr. Robinson draws attention to the psychological concommitants of chronic pelvic pain syndromes (e.g., decreased involvement with work and social activities, relationship problems, and sleep disturbances), while not ignoring possible organic bases (e.g., endometriosis). Of particular note is the incidence of depression— " . . . it is not clear whether the depression causes the pain or is a consequence of living with chronic pain."

He also comments on the contradictory evidence linking chronic pelvic pain syndrome with past sexual trauma, and that this syndrome can (but does not always) create marital sexual distress.

He strongly supports a multidisciplinary approach, and avoiding arguing with the patient as to whether there is an organic cause for the pain.

COMMENTARY

This brief report is yet another plea for an integrated, open-minded approach to the various chronic pain syndromes.

Smythe, H. A., Bennett, R. M., and Wolfe, F. (1993) Recognizing Fibromyalgia. *Patient Care*, March: pp. 53–72.

The authors describe fibromyalgia as the third most prevalent rheumatologic disorder, after osteo- and rheumatoid arthritis. They stress that the diagnostic criteria of pain in at least 11 of 18 trigger points will not allow confusion with any other disorder. They refer to stage-4, non-REM sleep disturbance, and suggest using small doses of tricyclic antidepressants to prevent the intrusion of alpha waves into stage-4 delta wave patterns. They point out that symptoms simulating fibromyalgia can be produced through sleep deprivation, thus emphasizing the importance of helping the patient achieve more normal and restorative sleep. They also refer to the frequency of association with irritable bowel syndrome, irritable bladder syndrome, chronic headache, and neurovascular instability, along with sensitivity to weather and environmental factors; and they also strongly suggest psychological testing such as the MMPI (Minnesota Multiphasic Personality Inventory) for all patients who suffer with chronic pain syndromes.

COMMENTARY

These authors differ somewhat in their estimation of the prevalence of fibromyalgia in the general population, estimating it to be only three to six percent. In most other ways, however, the two papers cited above are in agreement and overlap considerably, which can provide comfortable reassurance, again, to the sufferer.

Talbot, J. D., Marrett, S., Evans, A. C., Meyer, E., Bushnell, M. C., and Duncan, G. H. (1992) Multiple representations of pain in human cerebral cortex. *Science*, 251: pp. 1355–1358.

In this research, the authors demonstrated that painful heat stimuli cause significant activation in specific areas of the brain, viz. the contralateral anterior cingulate, secondary somatosensory, and primary sensory cortices. Furthermore, they state, the activation of the cingulate, unilaterally, indicates that this area of the forebrain, which is part of the limbic system and believed to regulate emotions, contains unexpectedly specific representations of pain.

This is an exceedingly detailed scientific article. The research is highly sophisticated, using a combination of PET (positron emission tomography) and MRI (magnetic resonance imaging) data in volunteer subjects as they were exposed to painful heat stimuli to the right forearm. Variables such as anxiety and emotional arousal were attended to by practice sessions and the determination for each subject of his/her level of noxious heat. Therefore, the administered stimuli were painfully hot but not unbearable.

The authors' conclusions were that ". . . the normal processing of painful stimuli in humans is not distributed over large areas of the cortex, but is restricted to three major structures—anterior cingulate cortex, S11, and S1. We propose that precise information about pain intensity reaches both parietal and frontal cortical areas. This information may then contribute to the evaluation of temporal and spatial features of pain in the parietal area and to the regulation of emotional reactions in the limbic regions of the frontal cortex."

COMMENTARY

This article can be gainfully considered in conjunction with the papers by Crawford, and Catchlove, all of which attend to the role of the limbic system and the implications for emotional involvement in chronic pain syndromes—something of which every patient and every clinician is exquisitely aware. The comments by Talbot et al. regarding the temporal and spatial features of pain are also reflective of the work by Katz and Melzack.

Some Concluding Comments

This cross-section of research and literature spans a wide spectrum—from newspaper reports to the most eminent medical and psychological journals. It is my hope that such a broad overview will give a sense of the diversity of research into chronic pain.

When preparing this section, I was struck by the way certain aspects were beginning to come together from a variety of sources—for instance those papers which detailed investigation into the limbic system, or the frequent pleas for a multidisciplinary approach.

It gives me hope that, as we learn more about the psychophysiology of these eroding, pervasive, sabotaging phenomena, there really will be more relief for those suffering from chronic pain.

For now, we are still struggling along, relying upon what we already have: the incredible ingenuity and resilience of the human psyche.

BIBLIOGRAPHY

Barber, J. & Adrian, C. (Eds.) *Psychological Approaches to the Management of Pain*. Brunner/Mazel, Publishers, New York, 1982.

Cousins, N. *Anatomy of an Illness (as Perceived by the Patient)*. W. W. Norton & Co., New York, 1979.

Donoghue, P. J. & Siegel, M. E. *Sick and Tired of Feeling Sick and Tired*. W. W. Norton & Co., New York, 1992.

Hall, H. *The Back Doctor: Lifetime Relief*. McLelland & Stewart, 1980.

Hall, H. *More Advice From the Back Doctor*. McLelland & Stewart, 1987.

Hilgard, R. H. & Hilgard, J. R. *Hypnosis in the Relief of Pain*. Wm. Kauffman, Inc., Los Altos, CA, 1975.

Hunter, M. E. *Psych Yourself In! Hypnosis and Health*. SeaWalk Press, West Vancouver, Canada, 1984, revised ed. 1987.

Hunter, M. E. *Creative Scripts for Hypnotherapy*. Brunner/Mazel, Inc., New York, 1994.

Levine, B. H. *Your Body Believes Every Word You Say*. Aslan Publishing, Lower Lake, CA, 1991.

Moyers, B. D. *Healing and the Mind*. Doubleday, New York, 1993.

Rose, L. *Overcoming Pain*. McCulloch Publishing Pty Ltd., Carlton, Victoria, Australia, 1990.

INDEX